Drugs and the Eye

Drugs and the Eye

Sponsored by the British Optical Association

Janet Vale, M.Sc., M.P.S.
Lecturer in Ocular Pharmacology,
University of Manchester

B. Cox, M.Sc., Ph.D., M.P.S.
Senior Lecturer in Pharmacology,
University of Manchester

BUTTERWORTHS
LONDON - BOSTON
Sydney - Wellington - Durban - Toronto

The Butterworth Group

United Kingdom — **Butterworth & Co (Publishers) Ltd**
London: 88 Kingsway, WC2B 6AB

Australia — **Butterworths Pty Ltd**
Sydney: 586 Pacific Highway, Chatswood, NSW 2067
Also at Melbourne, Brisbane, Adelaide and Perth

Canada — **Butterworth & Co (Canada) Ltd**
Toronto: 2265 Midland Avenue, Scarborough,
Ontario, M1P 4S1

New Zealand — **Butterworths of New Zealand Ltd**
Wellington: 26–28 Waring Taylor Street, 1

South Africa — **Butterworth & Co (South Africa) (Pty) Ltd**
Durban: 152–154 Gale Street

USA — **Butterworth (Publishers) Inc**
Boston: 19 Cummings Park, Woburn, Mass. 01801

First published 1978

ISBN 0 407 00128 X

British Library Cataloguing in Publication Data

Vale, M J
Drugs and the eye.
1. Therapeutics, Ophthalmological 2. Pharmacology
I. Title II. Cox, Barry, b.1937
617.7'061 RE991 77-30030

ISBN 0–407–00128–X

Typeset and produced by Scribe Design, Chatham , Kent
Printed in England by Butler & Tanner Ltd, Frome, Somerset

Preface

This book is concerned with all aspects of drug action in the eye which are of relevance to the ophthalmic optician or optometrist. It contains a concise discussion of relevant ocular anatomy and physiology so that the actions and uses of drugs may be put on a rational basis. The major groups of drugs used by the ophthalmic optician are discussed in detail and each section includes a discussion of the practical aspects of drug use. The groups of drugs covered include: cycloplegics, mydriatics, miotics, local anaesthetics, staining agents, antimicrobial agents, decongestants, antihistamines and anti-inflammatory agents. There are separate chapters dealing with first aid and emergency measures and with the legal aspects of the sale and supply of drugs commonly used in the eye. At the time of going to press some of the Acts covering the sale and supply of drugs are being repealed and replaced by new Acts. However, it is not expected that the changes will significantly modify the requirements placed on the ophthalmic optician.

A chapter on the ocular effects of drugs used systemically contains details not only of the ocular effects of named drugs but also of the conditions for which these drugs are likely to be used. There is a section on the solutions used in contact lens work, which deals both with the drugs used by the ophthalmic optician during fitting and those used by the patient in lens care. In each chapter the official (BP or BPC) preparations are listed and there is a section on the formulation of preparations for the eye. The physico-chemical properties underlying the absorption of drugs through the cornea are expanded so that the rationale behind the choice of a particular drug form and formulation may be understood.

As a whole, the book is designed to be a detailed yet concise account of drugs and their use in the eye.

It is intended that this book should be a working guide for qualified ophthalmic opticians/optometrists. However, since it contains considerable discussion not only of the practical aspects of drug use in the eye but also of the basic principles underlying this use, it should be invaluable to students reading for a degree or diploma in ophthalmic optics and optometry. As the book contains a detailed account of drug action in the eye and information on the diagnostic techniques it should be of value to the medical and allied professions. In this context it should be of interest to students of medicine, physiology, pharmacy, and pharmacology and also to nurses.

M.J.V.
B.C.

Contents

1

Anatomy and Physiology

A horizontal section through the eye is shown in *Figure 1.1*. There are three layers which enclose the transparent media through which light passes before reaching the retina.

The outer layer is protective in function. It is predominantly white in colour and opaque (the sclera) with a transparent anterior portion (the cornea).

The middle layer is mainly vascular and is made up of the choroid, ciliary body and iris. The innermost layer is the retina – predominantly nervous tissue. Within the three coats the eye is divided into two sections by the lens. The frontal section contains the aqueous humour, and is itself divided into anterior and posterior chambers by the iris. The section behind the lens contains the vitreous humour.

The important sites for drug action are the iris and ciliary muscle, the blood vessels, the extra-ocular muscles and the lacrimal gland (*Figure 1.2*). The iris and ciliary body are essentially composed of smooth muscle units which are innervated by the autonomic nervous system. The blood vessels and the levator palpebrae also contain smooth muscle units. Other extra-ocular muscles (for example, the recti and obliques) consist of striated muscle innervated by the somatic nervous system. The secretory cells of the lacrimal gland are innervated by both branches of the autonomic nervous system.

THE IRIS

The iris is a forward extension of the choroid and arises from the anterior face of the ciliary body. The pupil forms a central aperture in

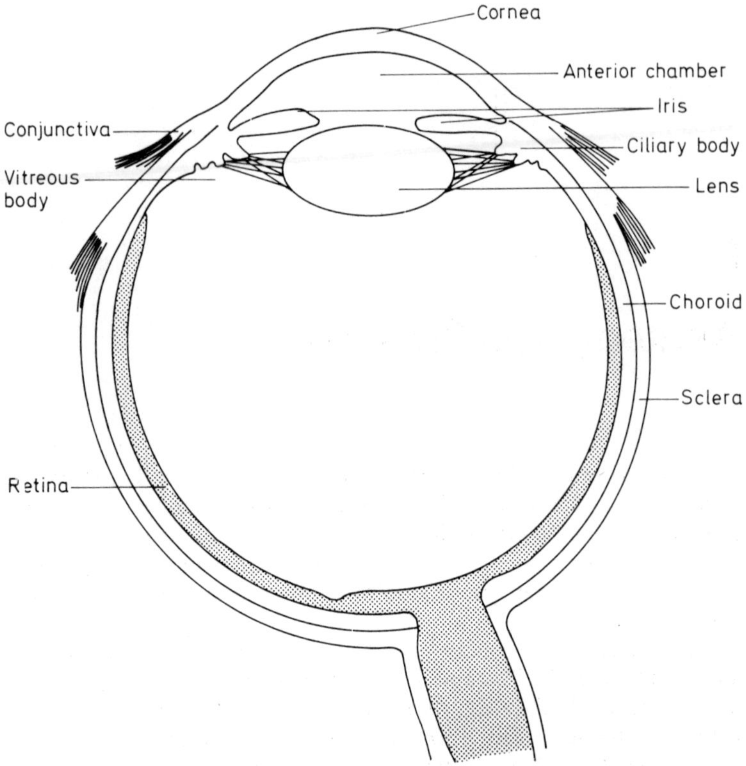

Figure 1.1 – A horizontal section through the eye

the iris. Two different muscle layers are contained within the iris tissue. These are the dilator pupillae and the sphincter pupillae. The dilator pupillae is made up of modified pigment epithelial cells which are arranged radially. These cells receive sympathetic innervation. Stimulation of this nerve supply produces a contraction of the cells resulting in an increase in pupil size (mydriasis). The sphincter pupillae is a typical smooth muscle structure with its fibres arranged in a circular fashion. It receives parasympathetic innervation. An increase in the activity of this nerve supply produces a contraction of the cells resulting in a decrease in pupil size (miosis), a decrease in the activity of this nerve supply allows a relaxation of the muscle cells resulting in an increase in pupil size (mydriasis).

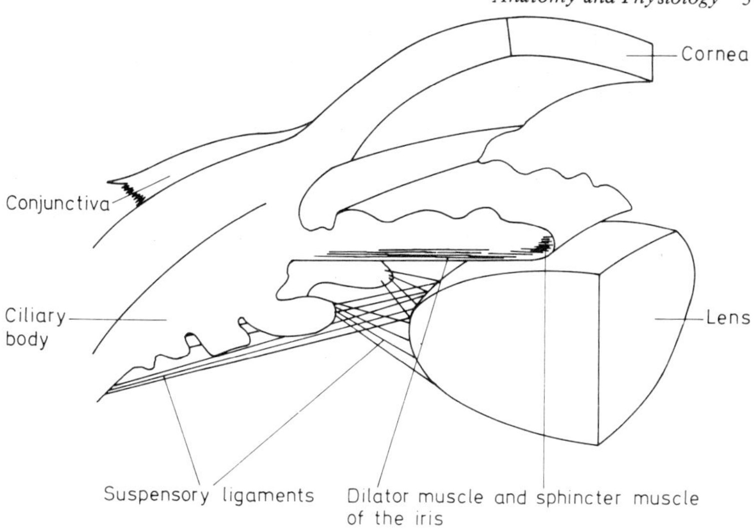

Figure 1.2 – Schematic diagram of the anterior chamber

THE CILIARY MUSCLE

The ciliary muscle is composed of smooth muscle units and is located against the inner surface of the anterior portion of the sclera. Most of the muscle fibres originate from the scleral region and run in meridional and radial groups. The innermost muscle fibres are arranged in the form of a sphincter and these receive parasympathetic innervation. Stimulation of the parasympathetic nerves causes contraction of the muscle, which in turn results in a lessening of the tension on the suspensory ligaments. This decrease in tension allows the lens to change shape, so that it becomes more convex. The change in the radius of curvature increases the power of the lens and allows near objects to be brought into focus at the retina.

INNERVATION OF THE IRIS AND CILIARY MUSCLE

The subdivision of the nervous system into central and peripheral components is shown in *Figure 1.3*.

The peripheral component is further subdivided into afferent or sensory neurones which carry impulses into the central nervous system, and efferent neurones which carry impulses out of the central nervous system. Efferent neurones may be either somatic, that is, those supplying skeletal muscle, or autonomic. The ciliary muscle and iris are innervated by the autonomic division.

There are two branches of the autonomic nervous system which are called parasympathetic and sympathetic. As can be seen in *Figures 1.4* and *1.5* the autonomic nerves supply most of the body's organs and tissues.

The iris receives both parasympathetic and sympathetic innervation. The parasympathetic nerve supply originates in the 3rd nerve nucleus in the central nervous system, which it leaves via the 3rd cranial nerve.

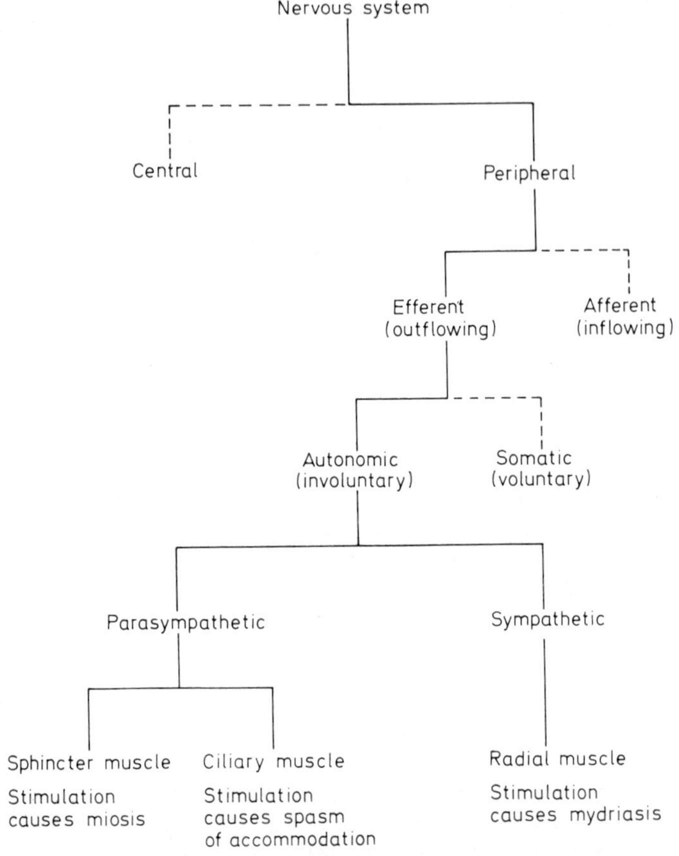

Figure 1.3 – Subdivision of the nervous system on an anatomical basis showing autonomic innervation of the eye

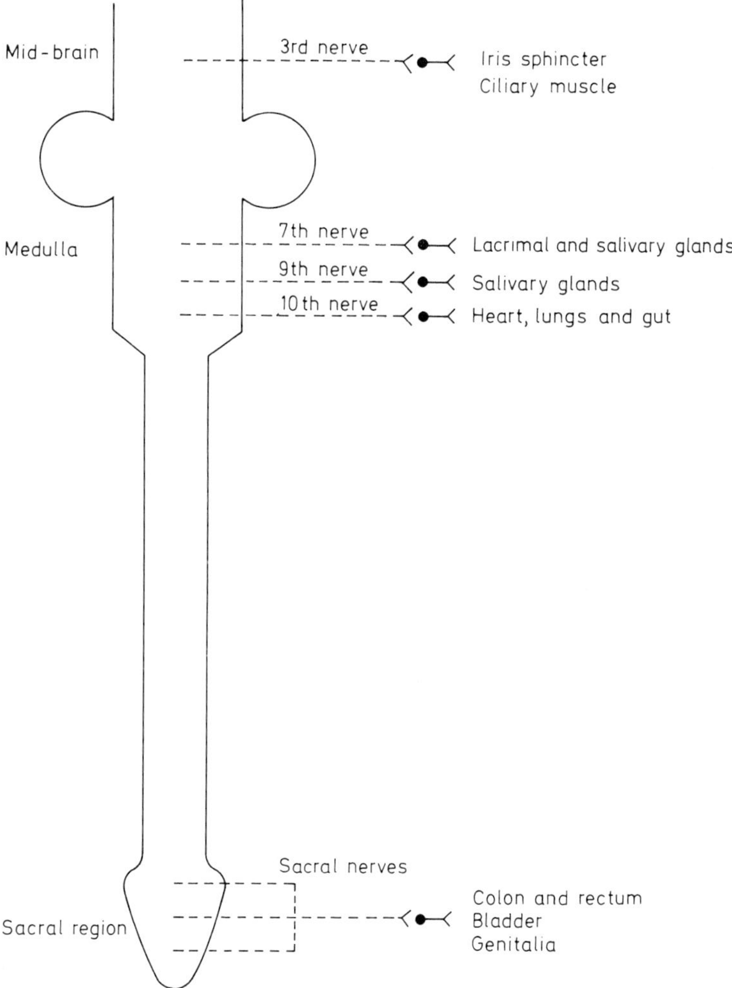

Figure 1.4 – The parasympathetic nervous system

There is a long preganglionic nerve which terminates in the ciliary ganglion (*Figure 1.6*). A short postganglionic fibre leaves the ganglion to innervate the sphincter pupillae. The lacrimal glands also receive parasympathetic nerves which originate in the 7th nerve nucleus and pass to the glands via the sphenopalatine ganglion. The sympathetic nerve supply leaves the spinal cord from the cervical and upper thoracic

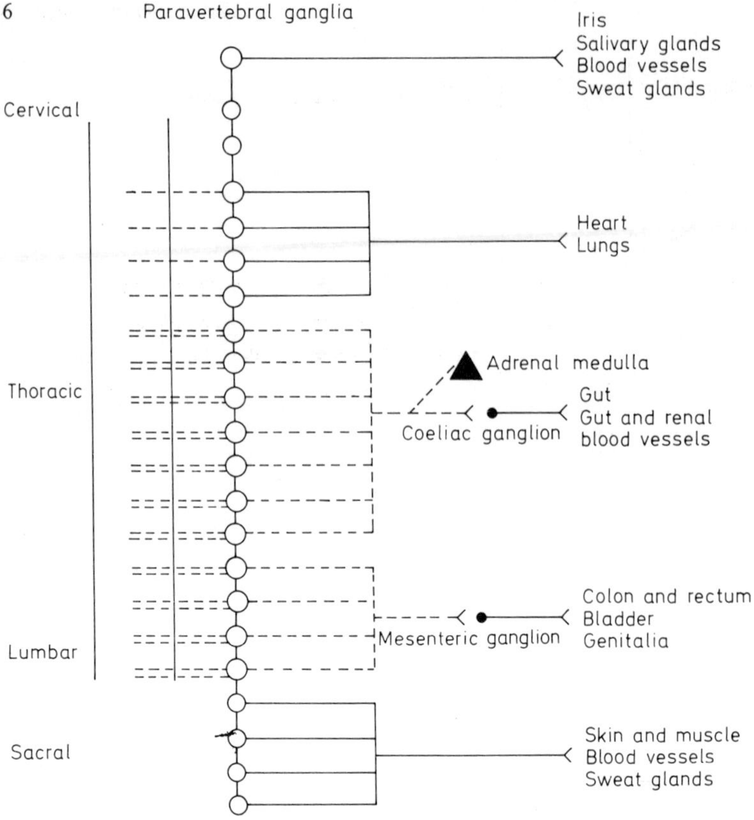

Paravertebral ganglia
Iris
Salivary glands
Blood vessels
Sweat glands
Cervical
Heart
Lungs
Adrenal medulla
Thoracic
Gut
Gut and renal
blood vessels
Coeliac ganglion
Colon and rectum
Bladder
Genitalia
Mesenteric ganglion
Lumbar
Skin and muscle
Blood vessels
Sweat glands
Sacral

Figure 1.5 – The sympathetic nervous system

SYMPATHETIC
PARASYMPATHETIC
Lacrimal gland
Lacrimal gland
Smooth muscle
of lid
Dilator
Sphincter
Sphenopalatine
ganglion
Superior
cervical
ganglion
7th nerve
Ciliary
muscle
Ciliary
ganglion
3rd nerve
Intermediate
ganglion
(see Figure 1.5)
Orbital
muscle

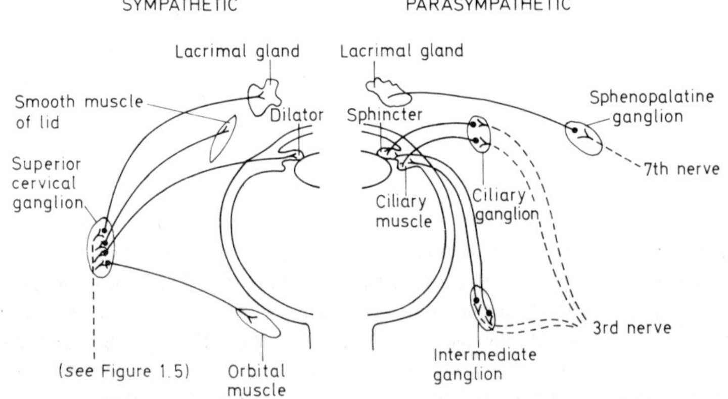

Figure 1.6 – Diagrammatic representation of the autonomic innervation of the eye

segments and ascends to the superior cervical ganglion where it terminates. A long postganglionic fibre which leaves the superior cervical ganglion then innervates the dilator pupillae muscle. Sympathetic postganglionic fibres from the superior cervical ganglion also innervate the lacrimal glands and the smooth muscle of the lids.

The effective nervous supply to the ciliary muscle is part of the parasympathetic system following a pathway similar to the nervous supply of the sphincter pupillae.

NEUROHUMOURAL TRANSMISSION AND THE RECEPTOR THEORY OF DRUG ACTION

It has been established in the previous section that the autonomic nervous system is composed of efferent pathways comprising two neurones, termed preganglionic and postganglionic, with a synapse between them. A synapse is the region of close approach between two neurones. At this site there is a small gap between the two which is called the synaptic cleft (20 nm). Thus, when a nerve impulse passes down a preganglionic fibre the impulse is not continuous in the postganglionic fibre. When the nerve impulse reaches the end of a preganglionic fibre it causes a chemical substance to be released. This diffuses across the synaptic cleft and comes into close contact with specially sensitive sites on the postganglionic neurone. The result of this close contact is alteration of the electrical properties of the postganglionic fibre and the initiation of a nerve impulse. A similar sequence of events occurs at the synapse between the postganglionic autonomic neurone and its effector cell (the neuro-effector junction) and also between a somatic motor neurone and a skeletal muscle cell (the neuromuscular junction). This process of chemical transmission of nerve impulses is known as neurohumoural transmission.

Two substances have been identified as chemical transmitters of peripheral nervous activity, they are acetylcholine and noradrenaline. Acetylcholine is the transmitter liberated from presynaptic nerves to act upon postsynaptic effector cells at the following four sites:

(1) All ganglia.
(2) At postganglionic parasympathetic nerve endings.
(3) At the skeletal neuromuscular junction.
(4) At a few postganglionic sympathetic nerve endings, that is, postganglionic sympathetic fibres concerned with sweating and with the dilatation of blood vessels of skeletal muscle.

Noradrenaline is a transmitter at postganglionic sympathetic nerve endings with the exception of the two areas listed under (4) above. Historically the transmitter was once thought to be adrenaline and these nerves are still referred to as adrenergic.

The following sequence of events takes place at all synapses:

(1) The transmitter is synthesized and stored in the nerve ending.
(2) Nerve impulses cause the release of the transmitter into the synaptic cleft.
(3) The transmitter diffuses across the gap and activates the sensitive postsynaptic area (receptor).
(4) The transmitter is rendered inactive.

SITES RECEIVING CHOLINERGIC INNERVATION

A diagrammatic representation of the sequence of events occurring at such a site is shown in *Figure 1.7.*

The chemical substance choline is concentrated within the presynaptic nerve ending by means of a specialized transport system known as the choline pump(1). This transport system requires energy and is susceptible to metabolic poisons. Once inside the nerve ending the choline combines with acetyl coenzyme A to form the ester acetylcholine (*Figure 1.7*). This reaction is catalysed by the enzyme choline acetylase(2).

The acetylcholine so formed is stored in specially differentiated parts of the nerve ending called vesicles(3). When a nerve impulse passes down the presynaptic neurone vesicular acetylcholine is released into the synaptic cleft(4) and diffuses to the postsynaptic site(5). After activating the receptor the acetycholine diffuses away and comes into contact with an enzyme, acetylcholinesterase(6). This enzyme is found predominantly in the synaptic regions and causes a reversal of the process depicted in (2). The choline so liberated is available for re-uptake into the presynaptic nerve for the synthesis of new transmitter material.

Drugs may interfere at various points in this sequence of events. The stages subject to drug interference and the types of drug active at these stages are shown in *Figure 1.8*.

Drugs such as hemicholinium will compete with choline for the choline pump(1) so that choline cannot gain access into the presynaptic nerve. This prevents synthesis of new transmitter material and eventual loss of transmission. Other drugs such as tri-ethylcholine are taken up

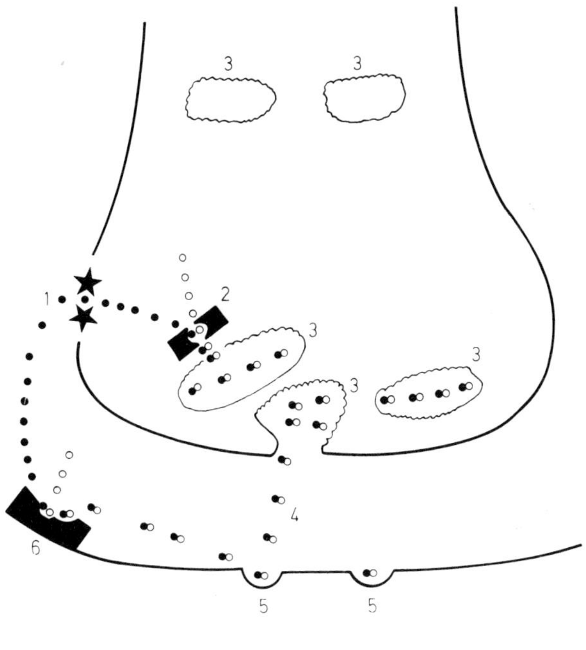

● ○ ●○

Choline + Acetyl coenzyme A = Acetylcholine + Coenzyme A

Figure 1.7 – Diagrammatic representation of cholinergic synapse showing synthesis, release and inactivation of acetylcholine (●○)

by the choline pump and compete with choline inside the nerve, resulting in the production of acetyltriethylcholine (2), which is stored in a similar way to acetylcholine (3). However, acetyltriethylcholine is relatively ineffective after release (4).

All the drugs mentioned above will act at any synapse at which acetylcholine is the transmitter and whilst they may be of value and interest to the pharmacologist or physiologist they are not of therapeutic value.

The next stage in neurotransmission is Stage (5), the process of transmitter receptor interaction. The drugs which act at this point in the sequence are of therapeutic value. Drugs acting like acetylcholine are called agonists (for example, pilocarpine), and those which prevent the action of acetylcholine by blocking access to the receptor are the

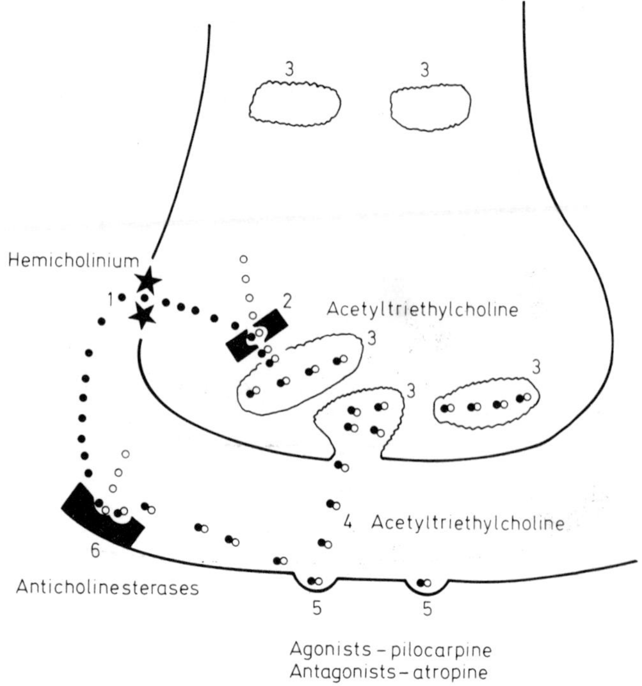

Figure 1.8 – Diagrammatic representation of the sites at which drugs may interfere with the functioning of a cholinergic synapse

antagonists (for example, atropine). The final stage in the sequence of events occurring at these synapses is the enzymatic breakdown of acetylcholine and this stage is also susceptible to drug interference. Thus, some drugs combine with the enzyme acetylcholinesterase (6) which is present in the synaptic cleft. These drugs, the anticholinesterases, interact with the active sites on the acetylcholinesterase but are not hydrolysed. They therefore prevent the access of acetylcholine to the enzyme and cause an increased concentration of acetylcholine in the synaptic cleft, thereby increasing the number of transmitter receptor interactions. Another family of cholinesterase enzymes also occurs in the body associated with serum and with muscle. These enzymes, often called pseudocholinesterases, will hydrolyse other esters and some amides as well as acetylcholine, and are also susceptible to attack by the anticholinesterases. The function of this group is probably to hydrolyse esters which either enter the body in the food, or occur as the result of metabolic processes.

In order to fully understand the interactions of drugs at receptor sites a more detailed description of the transmitter receptor interaction is required. It is postulated that the interaction between acetylcholine and the receptor relies on the physico-chemical properties of the transmitter substance and the receptor site. Thus, acetylcholine in solution can be regarded as a carbon skeleton, which is neutral, carrying chemical substituents which bear small electrical charges. As shown in *Figure 1.9*

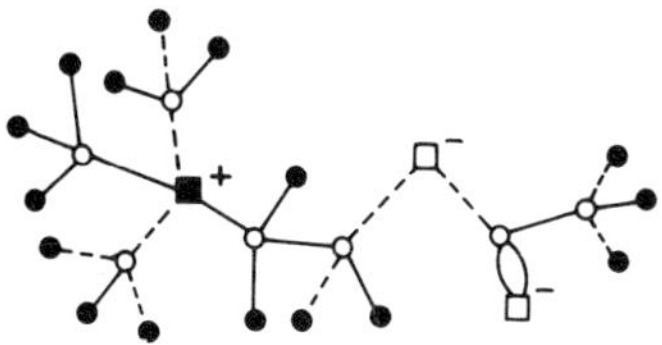

● Hydrogen atom

○ Carbon atom

■ Nitrogen atom

□ Oxygen atom

Figure 1.9 – Chemical structure of the acetylcholine molecule to show the probable distribution of the electropositive (+) and electronegative (–) charges

a small positive charge resides on the nitrogen and small negative charges on the oxygen substituents. The receptor similarly will carry small electrical charges distributed in such a way that the negative charges of the transmitter correspond to the positive charges of the receptor and the positive charges of the transmitter correspond to the negative charges of the receptor. When these two come into contact the resulting interaction causes changes in the structure of the receptor. It is these changes which initiate a sequence of events such as nerve action potential or muscle contraction. Acetylcholine is not a rigid structure and may exist in solution in many conformations. Whilst one particular conformation may be satisfactory for interaction with, say, a receptor on a nerve (that is, at a ganglion) this conformation will not necessarily be suitable for interaction with the receptor on a skeletal muscle or on an autonomic effector cell. Therefore, whilst acetylcholine is the transmitter at all these sites it is postulated that the receptors differ. Because of this fact it is possible to select drugs which have a specific action on one type of receptor. The prime example of such a drug is the alkaloid muscarine. Thus, this drug has a similar configuration to that of acetylcholine when acetylcholine interacts with the autonomic effector cells innervated by postganglionic parasympathetic nerves. It is therefore selective for the receptors on these cells and has led to their description as muscarinic receptors. Muscarine does not have the same configuration as acetylcholine when this latter substance acts in the ganglia or on a skeletal muscle receptor. Another alkaloid, nicotine, has some structural similarity to the conformation of acetylcholine when it acts at these other two sites. Thus, these receptors are classified as nicotinic receptors.

DRUG ACTION AT THE MUSCARINIC RECEPTOR

This may be subdivided into drugs which interact with the receptor to produce an effect similar to acetylcholine and those which interact with the receptor but do not produce those changes which are associated with an acetylcholine interaction. However, by virtue of the drug occupation of receptor sites, access of acetylcholine is prevented and transmission at the site is blocked. Drugs acting like acetylcholine at the receptor are called muscarinic agonists, for example, pilocarpine; drugs blocking the action of acetylcholine at the receptor are called muscarinic antagonists, for example, atropine, homatropine and cyclopentolate. Thus, the muscarinic agonists will act on the ciliary muscle and sphincter pupillae to cause spasm of accommodation and miosis. Muscarinic antagonists will act at these sites to produce paralysis of accommodation (cycloplegia) and mydriasis.

DRUG ACTION AT THE NICOTINIC RECEPTORS

Receptors for acetylcholine are similar in all ganglia whether sympathetic or parasympathetic. However, the nicotinic receptor at the ganglion is not identical with the nicotinic receptor at the neuromuscular junction. The evidence for this statement is based on the fact that some drugs will interact with the ganglion receptors to prevent the action of acetylcholine but are relatively ineffective at the receptors on skeletal muscle. Hexamethonium and pempidine are efficient ganglion blocking agents but do not cause muscle paralysis. Drugs such as tubocurarine and decamethonium are potent antagonists at skeletal muscle receptors, causing muscle paralysis, but they are relatively ineffective in blocking the ganglion receptors. The effects of ganglion blockade are complex because many tissues are innervated by both sympathetic and parasympathetic nerves and therefore the end result depends on the relative importance of the two systems. Since the parasympathetic system is dominant in the iris and ciliary muscle the ocular effects of ganglion blockade are mydriasis and cycloplegia. Drugs with blocking actions at the nicotinic receptors in skeletal muscle are not used by the ophthalmic optician but are reserved primarily to produce muscular relaxation in surgery or electro-convulsive therapy.

SITES RECEIVING ADRENERGIC INNERVATION

A diagrammatic representation of the sequence of events at an adrenergic synapse is shown in *Figure 1.10*.

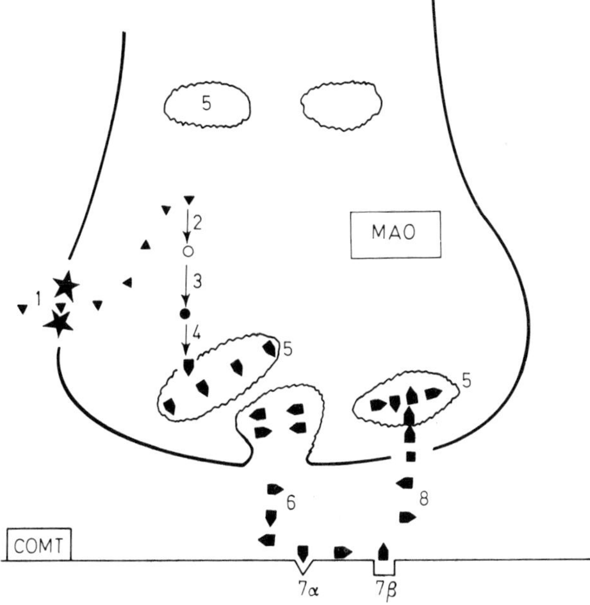

Figure 1.10 – Diagrammatic representation of an adrenergic synapse showing the synthesis, release and inactivation of noradrenaline (⯆)

The amino acid tyrosine (1) is taken up by the presynaptic nerve. Once inside the nerve a sequence of enzymatic steps take place (2–4) leading to the formation of noradrenaline which is concentrated in granulated vesicles (5) present in the nerve endings. When a nerve impulse reaches the terminal the stored noradrenaline is released into the synaptic cleft (6) and diffuses to the postsynaptic receptor site (7, α or β). After interaction with the receptor site (often called the adrenoceptor) the noradrenaline diffuses back across the synaptic cleft and is actively taken up into the presynaptic neurone (8). This uptake process is energy dependent, saturable and relatively specific. The number of transmitter receptor interactions is related to the concentration of the transmitter in the area of the receptor. Thus, when noradrenaline is removed from the synaptic cleft and concentrated within the nerve the number of transmitter receptor interactions declines and the transmitter effect is reduced and eventually abolished. This mechanism is the major one involved in the inactivation of noradrenaline.

There are two enzymes in the body capable of metabolizing noradrenaline, these are monoamine oxidase (MAO) and catechol-o-methyl transferase (COMT). However, these are not important for the inactivation of noradrenaline released from the presynaptic nerve. Large quantities of monoamine oxidase are found in the liver where its function is to metabolize naturally occurring amines present in the blood stream. It is also present in nerves and it oxidizes a proportion of the intraneuronal noradrenaline which is not in the vesicle. Catechol-o-methyl transferase occurs mainly within the effector cells and in the liver and kidney. It is an enzyme of low specificity and has other substrates.

The points at which drugs may interfere with the sequence are shown in *Figure 1.11*.

The various steps in the synthetic pathway of noradrenaline are subject to inhibition leading to a decreased production of the natural transmitter and loss of transmission. Alpha-methyldopa (1) is a compound capable of entering the synthetic pathway. Alpha-methylnoradrenaline is produced rather than noradrenaline (2–4). The alpha-methyl compound is stored (5) and released in the same way as noradrenaline but it is much less effective at the postsynaptic receptor site. Thus, transmission of the impulse is inhibited. Release of noradrenaline following a nerve impulse may be blocked by a group of drugs known as adrenergic neurone blocking agents (6). These compounds, which include guanethidine, bethanidine and bretylium, appear to concentrate in the fine endings of postganglionic sympathetic nerves and thereby interfere with the release process. Alpha-methyldopa and the adrenergic neurone blocking agents are used to reduce sympathetic activity in an attempt to combat hypertension. Other drugs act postsynaptically interfering with transmitter receptor interactions. There are at least two types of receptor found at the postganglionic sympathetic nerve effector cell junction. These two receptors are designated α and β (7). In general, interaction between the transmitter

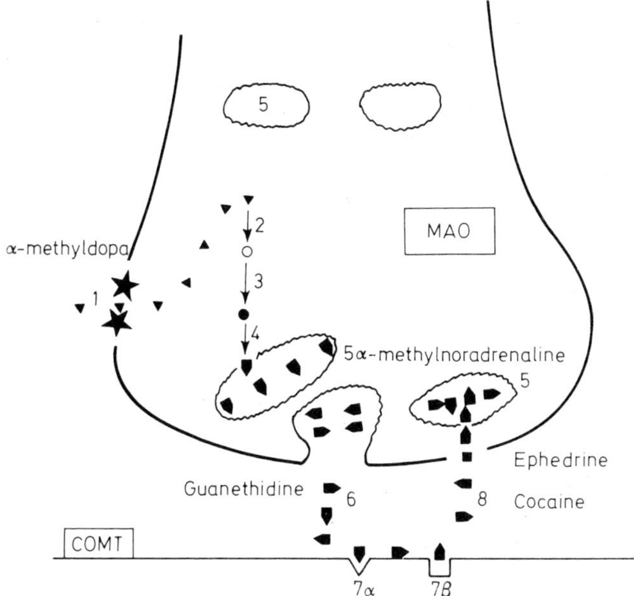

Figure 1.11 – Diagrammatic representation of the sites at which drugs may interfere with the functioning of an adrenergic synapse

and an α receptor causes an excitatory response, for example, contraction of the smooth muscle cells of the dilator pupillae, and interaction between the transmitter and a β receptor causes an inhibitory response. The exception to this is that interaction with the β receptors in the heart results in increased rate and force of contraction. Noradrenaline is predominantly active at the α receptors. Adrenaline, the hormone synthesized and stored in the adrenal medulla and released into the blood stream in response to stress, has approximately equal activity at both types of receptors. There are a large number of synthetic compounds which have sufficient structural resemblance to the natural transmitter to be able to interact with either of the receptor types and produce a response. Amongst these compounds with agonist activity are phenylephrine (7 α) which acts almost exclusively with α adrenoceptors and isoprenaline (7 β) which acts almost exclusively with β adrenoceptors. Phenylephrine and isoprenaline are known as directly acting sympathomimetics. Certain compounds, for example, ephedrine have some direct action but the major part of their activity is indirect. Thus, they penetrate the neurone (8) enter the vesicular store and cause noradrenaline to be released (6) into the synaptic cleft. The released noradrenaline is available for interaction with the receptor. As was stated earlier the most important factor in decreasing transmitter receptor interactions is the active re-uptake of noradrenaline into the nerve endings. A number of drugs, including cocaine, are able to block this active process (8) and thus maintain a higher concentration of noradrenaline in the vicinity of the receptor. Use of either type of indirectly acting drug will result in increased sympathetic activity, for example, contraction of the dilator pupillae.

A second type of effect on transmitter receptor interactions is possible. This is an inhibition of transmitter receptor interactions. There are some drugs which bear sufficient structural resemblance to noradrenaline to interact with the receptors but after combination with the receptor produce no response (antagonists). The presence of the antagonist means that the number of transmitter receptor interactions is reduced because noradrenaline cannot gain access to the receptor. These antagonists at the adrenoceptors are divided into two types depending on whether they block either α receptors (phenoxybenzamine,phentolamine, 7α) or β receptors (propranolol, 7β). These compounds are not of direct practical importance to the ophthalmic optician.

2

Factors Affecting Drug Absorption

The drugs used by the ophthalmic optician are usually applied to the eye in the form of drops or, more rarely, ointments. Topical application is used in order to restrict the site of drug action to the eye, reduce the possibility of unwanted systemic effects and reduce the quantity of drug employed. However, in order to achieve this localized action there must be sufficient absorption from the site of application to give and maintain effective drug concentrations at the site of action. The absorptive surface in question is the cornea. Any drug absorbed by the conjunctiva enters the systemic circulation and is lost from the eye. Drug loss may also occur through the puncta unless pressure is placed on the nasal canthus. The cornea consists essentially of three parts: the epithelium, the stroma and the endothelium. The epithelium and the endothelium both have a high lipid content and are therefore readily penetrated by compounds with high lipid solubility (that is, non-polar, non-charged structures). The stroma lying between the epithelium and endothelium is an aqueous structure containing some 75–80 per cent water. This layer will therefore be more readily penetrated by compounds which are polar and water-soluble (for example, ionized particles). In order for a drug placed on the cornea to penetrate all three parts of the cornea it must therefore be both lipid and water-soluble. Hydrocarbon structures confer lipid solubility on a compound, water solubility depends on the presence of hydrophilic or polar moieties such as hydroxyl (OH) or ionized groups in the structure. A structure containing only hydrocarbon groupings will exhibit high lipid solubility and poor water solubility. A compound having polar substituents will show high water solubility and poor lipid solubility. In either of these extreme cases the compound would not be capable of crossing all the layers of the cornea. A compound whose structure contains both some non-polar and some polar groupings will show both lipid and water solubility and will therefore be able to cross the cornea.

The majority of drugs used by the optician are weak bases. A weak base is employed as its water-soluble acid salt, for example, ephedrine hydrochloride (*Figure 2.1a*). Thus, in solution this will exist in both the ionized (water-soluble) and unionized (lipid-soluble) forms in equilibrium according to *Figure 2.1b* and satisfy the above criteria for corneal

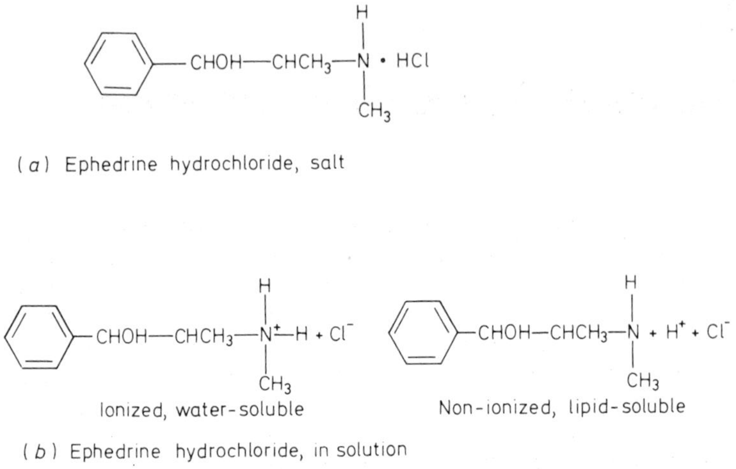

$$C_6H_5\text{—CHOH—CHCH}_3\text{—N(H)(CH}_3\text{)} \cdot HCl$$

(*a*) Ephedrine hydrochloride, salt

$$C_6H_5\text{—CHOH—CHCH}_3\text{—}\overset{+}{N}(CH_3)\text{—}H + Cl^- \qquad C_6H_5\text{—CHOH—CHCH}_3\text{—N(H)(CH}_3) + H^+ + Cl^-$$

Ionized, water-soluble — Non-ionized, lipid-soluble

(*b*) Ephedrine hydrochloride, in solution

Figure 2.1 – Dissociation of ephedrine hydrochloride (a weak base) in aqueous solution

penetration. (For a more detailed discussion of the factors affecting the absorption of a weak base *see* Appendix.)

Some synthetic drugs are quaternary amines and highly ionized in solution at any pH. Thus, they have poor lipid solubility and poor penetration of the cornea (for example, neostigmine, and carbachol). Surface active agents, such as benzalkonium chloride, which reduce surface tension are able to increase the permeability of the cornea and aid penetration by drugs. Benzalkonium chloride may be used for this purpose with carbachol (a muscarinic agonist) or neostigmine (an anticholinesterase).

As the absorption is a passive process an important factor for absorption is the concentration gradient. In passive absorption drugs diffuse down a concentration gradient from an area of high concentration. Solutions employed by opticians are relatively concentrated. The concentration in the aqueous humour or tissues of the eye does not approach that in the solution and provides no hindrance to absorption.

Eye drops have often been formulated to be isotonic but it seems that variations from isotonicity do no great harm to the eye. Hypertonicity may cause stinging and hypotonicity may increase the permeability of the cornea.

Another factor which may influence the absorption of drugs is damage to the corneal tissues. Removal or abrasion of the epithelium can increase the absorption of drugs with low lipid solubility (although the endothelium must still be crossed). This may lead to unexpectedly high concentrations of drugs in the eye.

One final consideration is the form in which the drug is presented to the eye – aqueous drops, oily drops or ointments. Aqueous drops are the presentation most commonly used. These are convenient to use but have the disadvantage of a short contact time with the cornea, and a short time for absorption. Rapid initial absorption is therefore important and it would be preferable for the drug to be as little ionized as possible. Unfortunately, as most drugs employed are the acid salts of weak bases, the major portion will be in the ionized form. As drops are often placed in the lower fornix a portion of the drug may be absorbed by the conjunctiva rather than the cornea and lost in the systemic circulation. Alternatively, some drug may be lost by passage through the puncta into the nose.

If oily drops or ointments are used the base is more likely to be in its unionized lipid-soluble form suitable for absorption across the epithelium. This, together with the longer contact time of an oily preparation would suggest that absorption would be more rapid, provided that the base was capable of ionizing in the aqueous stroma. One possible disadvantage is that the drug may be more soluble in the oily base of the ointment than in the lipid layer of the cornea and therefore be trapped in the ointment.

3

Cycloplegics

A cycloplegic drug causes paralysis of accommodation. It thus renders the eye unable to focus on near objects and does this by inhibiting the effect of acetylcholine released from postganglionic parasympathetic nerves. Atropine is a typical example of this class of drug. Atropine competes with acetylcholine for the receptor sites on smooth muscle, in this case on the ciliary body. The action of acetylcholine is thus prevented, the ciliary muscle is not responsive to parasympathetic nerve activity and relaxes. The tension on the suspensory ligaments of the lens is increased so that the lens itself becomes less convex and accommodation is inhibited.

Atropine and atropine-like drugs do not affect nerve impulses, neither do they prevent the release of acetylcholine.

As the sphincter pupillae also has postganglionic parasympathetic innervation the constrictor action of acetylcholine at this site is also antagonized and the pupil dilates. With this group of drugs cycloplegia is always accompanied by mydriasis.

Atropine

Atropine is a naturally occurring alkaloid extracted from various Solanaceous plants including *Atropa belladonna* (deadly nightshade) and *Datura stramonium* (thorn apple). It is an organic ester formed by the combination of an aromatic acid and an organic base tropine (*Figure 3.1*).

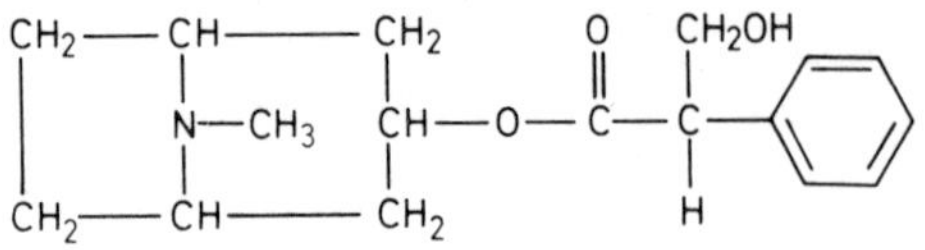

Figure 3.1 – Structure of atropine

MODE OF ACTION

Atropine is a competitive antagonist of acetylcholine. That is to say, the drug atropine and the transmitter acetylcholine are in direct competition with each other for the acetylcholine muscarinic receptor sites on smooth muscle. If acetylcholine occupies the receptor then a sequence of events occur resulting in muscle contraction. If atropine occupies the receptor this is not available to acetylcholine, the sequence is prevented and the muscle is relaxed. Two factors are important in determining the number of receptors occupied by a drug. First, the affinity of the drug for the receptor and, secondly, the concentration of the drug in the tissue fluid surrounding the receptor (the biophase). Atropine has a high affinity for the muscarinic receptor and therefore is effective in relatively low concentrations and its effects are long lived and difficult to reverse.

ACTIONS IN THE EYE

Sphincter pupillae

After instillation of a 1 per cent solution of atropine sulphate mydriasis usually commences within 10–15 minutes and the maximum effect is reached within 30–40 minutes. At this time the pupil is widely dilated and the response to light is abolished. The return to normal pupil size is slow and may take several days (up to 10 days).

Ciliary muscle

As the ciliary muscle lies deeper in the eye than the sphincter pupillae the diffusion path of the drug is longer. Therefore the onset of cycloplegia is later than the onset of mydriasis. A slight decrease in accommodation may be noted within 30 minutes. The decrease in amplitude progresses slowly, a maximum effect occurring in 1–3 hours. Some recovery from the cycloplegic effect of atropine begins in 2–3 days. The ability to read fine print has usually returned in 3 days but recovery of full amplitude of accommodation may take up to 10 days.

Secretions

Atropine reduces the secretory activity of the salivary, gastro-intestinal, lacrimal and sweat glands. Its effect on the lacrimal gland is of interest because it alters the character of the secretion, reducing its water content and thereby increasing the concentration of solutes. Tear fluid contains an enzyme, lysosyme, which is active against a number of bacteria by an action on their cell walls. Atropine will increase the concentration of lysosyme in lacrimal fluid, thus increasing its anti-bacterial properties.

Intra-ocular pressure

There is a possibility that the use of atropine may lead to an increase in intra-ocular pressure. Dilation of the pupil will result in the iris being thickened and 'piled up' in the angle of the anterior chamber. In the case of a shallow anterior chamber the outflow of fluid through the trabecular meshwork, the canal of Schlemm and the aqueous veins may be hindered. The alternate contractions and relaxations of the ciliary muscle during normal accommodation exert a varying pull on the scleral spur and have some effect in changing the size of, and pressure within, the canal. If pressure increases then fluid passes more easily into the intra-scleral veins than back into the anterior chamber. If the pressure falls in the canal then fluid will pass into the canal from the anterior chamber, but will not be drawn back from the intra-scleral veins which have valves to prevent this happening. Thus, normal movements of the ciliary muscle during accommodation produce a pumping action aiding outflow of fluid from the eye. Atropine will prevent this action, again tending to reduce outflow. Other factors which have been postulated to contribute to the increase in intra-ocular pressure after atropine are:

(1) Facilitated inflow and impeded outflow of blood due to the immobilization of the ciliary muscle. This may result in intra-ocular congestion.

(2) An increase in capillary permeability possibly by a mechanism involving histamine release.

The above considerations pose the question: why is it that atropine does not always produce an increase in intra-ocular pressure? The answer lies in the efficient regulatory mechanisms which the normal eye can bring into play. As pressure rises the outflow of aqueous increases and the rate of aqueous secretion decreases. This will tend to keep intra-ocular pressure constant. However, with increased age changes take place in the eye which reduce the efficiency of the regulatory mechanisms.

(1) The sclera becomes less distensible by losing its elastic properties. Any increase in intra-ocular congestion will thus produce a relatively greater effect on the pressure.

(2) Bundles of fibres at the filtration angle become sclerosed and thickened, thus impeding outflow.

(3) Pigment from the iris and the ciliary body becomes trapped and collects between the fibres impeding outflow.

(4) The lens increases in size, both in thickness and in diameter. The space between the periphery of the lens and the ciliary processes is decreased, the iris is pushed forward producing a shallow anterior chamber and a narrowing of the angle.

In many people these changes do not exceed certain critical limits and therefore there is no increase in intra-ocular pressure. In other people the changes occur to an unusual degree, particularly in the hyperopic eye (small globe, normal lens and large ciliary muscle). In these people there is a tendency towards an increased intra-ocular pressure and under the stresses induced by atropine treatment an attack of glaucoma can ensue.

Thus, the use of atropine in older people can be very dangerous and as it would be of little or no benefit in the refraction of this age group its use should be rigorously avoided.

OTHER ACTIONS OF ATROPINE

The pharmacological basis of the use of atropine as a cycloplegic and mydriatic has been discussed. The parasympathetic nervous system innervates a wide variety of tissues. Therefore a blocking drug such as atropine will bring about a number of other actions if sufficient is absorbed following topical application or if the drug is ingested.

The heart

Atropine will produce an increase in heart rate. The heart rate is determined by two separate factors, a sympathetic innervation which acts to produce an increase and a parasympathetic innervation (the vagus nerve) which causes a decrease. Atropine will block the effect of acetylcholine released from the vagus nerve resulting in a decrease in vagal tone and an increase in heart rate. This increase after atropine is usually more pronounced in children who have a higher vagal tone.

The circulation

In usual therapeutic doses atropine has little effect on the blood pressure as most vascular tissue is without parasympathetic innervation. High doses of atropine may cause a fall in blood pressure but this is most likely mediated by an action on the central nervous system. Atropine may also cause dilatation in cutaneous blood vessels which is most prominent in the blush area. It is thought likely that this effect is due to release of histamine.

Smooth muscle

Atropine will reduce the tone and motility of most smooth muscle tissue although some tissues with parasympathetic innervation, for example, the bladder, are more resistant to atropine than others. Both the tone and motility of the gastro-intestinal tract are decreased as is the tone and motility in the ureters. The smooth muscles of the bronchioles are also relaxed giving a slight decrease in airway resistance.

Secretions

Atropine will produce a reduction in the secretions of a number of glands with postganglionic parasympathetic innervation, for example, salivary glands, mucous secreting glands of the bronchioles and gastro-intestinal tract. Secretion of gastric acid is less affected by atropine as this is mainly under hormonal control. Atropine also reduces sweating. The eccrine sweat glands of the skin are innervated by postganglionic sympathetic nerve fibres. These fibres differ from other postganglionic sympathetic nerves in that the transmitter released is acetylcholine not noradrenaline.

Central effects

In very low doses atropine stimulates the central nervous system. Stimulation of the medulla and higher cerebral centres results in stimulation of respiration and slowing of the heart due to an action on vagal centres. This occurs before the concentration of atropine in peripheral tissues reaches a sufficient level to antagonize the acetylcholine released from postganglionic cholinergic nerves. Some slight agitation and excitement may be observed.

If the dose of atropine is progressively increased these effects become more prominent developing through restlessness, irritability, disorientation and hallucinations to delirium. At very high doses the effect of atropine on the central nervous system changes to a depressant action and death ensues due to respiratory paralysis.

Atropine as a poison

Atropine poisoning due to absorption of the drug from ocular membranes or after passage through the puncta and subsequent absorption is a possibility. There have been some reports of psychotic changes and alterations in heart rate after the use of 1 per cent atropine sulphate eye drops. These cases have led to the suggestion that if drops are to be used in children under the age of 7 years the concentration should not exceed 0.5 per cent. The main danger from atropine is likely to be the accidental ingestion of the preparation, the ointment most often being supplied for use at home under the supervision of the parent.

The symptoms and signs of atropine poisoning are very typical, being a mixture of central and peripheral actions. They include dry mouth causing difficulty in swallowing and speaking, and thirst, nausea and vomiting, rapid respiration, dilated pupils, fixed blurred vision, photophobia, a hot dry flushed skin, high temperature and a rapid pulse. The patient becomes very restless and excited, he may become confused and suffer hallucinations. Motor incoordination ensues and the central excitation changes to central depression. Respiration becomes inadequate and ultimately leads to coma and death from respiratory depression.

It is perhaps a sobering thought that deaths in children have resulted from as little as 10 mg of atropine although in some cases there has been recovery from as much as 1 g. A tube of eye ointment containing 3 g of a 1 per cent preparation would contain 30 mg of atropine sulphate.

Atropine irritation

This is a local reaction of the tissues shown only in a few patients who are hypersensitive to the drug. It is an allergic response requiring prior sensitization. Thus, the response does not appear the first time the drug is used, but only on subsequent occasions. The first step in the sensitization process is the combination of atropine with some substance which occurs naturally in the body. This substance, which is probably a protein, has antigenic properties. The antigen then induces the formation of antibodies (similar to those produced in response to an infection) by the plasma cells. The antibodies become attached to special cells in the body called mast cells. The mast cells are widely distributed throughout the body and are basophilic granular cells found in loose connective tissues and the peripheral blood. They have a high histamine, heparin and 5-hydroxytryptamine content. An allergic response requires antibody-antigen interaction. On the first exposure to atropine the antibody is produced. However, during the formation of the antibody the concentration of atropine in the body is already declining due to metabolism and excretion. Therefore the relative concentrations of antibody and antigen are not optimal for interaction and no allergic response results.

On a second application of the drug the antibody levels rise much more rapidly and an interaction does take place. The reaction is thought to take place at the mast cell surface where the antibody is bound, an intracellular enzyme is activated, which in turn causes the release of histamine, 5-hydroxytryptamine, a substance known as slow reacting substance (SRS) and various kinins. Although all these substances have been implicated in the allergic response histamine appears to be the major active component. Histamine causes capillary dilatation and increased capillary permeability. This therefore leads to a warming of the skin and an area of oedema (collection of fluid within the tissue but outside the vascular system). A second action of histamine mediated through local nerve reflexes is to cause arteriolar vasodilatation. The affected area and surrounding tissue becomes red and hot. Itching is added to the already considerable discomfort. Thus, if atropine irritation were to occur after a second or later instillation the skin round the eye would appear red and inflamed with swelling of the lids and conjunctiva. The conjunctiva would also appear red and inflamed and the patient would complain of itching and irritation. The condition frequently spreads to the upper nasal mucous membranes.

Although this condition is relatively rare and often only occurs after prolonged treatment with atropine (as in iritis) it is a condition of which the optician should be aware. The immediate and essential step when the allergic response occurs is withdrawal of the drug. If continued use of a cycloplegic is essential then some other compound must be substituted, preferably one with a chemical structure which is not closely related to the atropine molecule (*Figure 3.2*). Thus, if homatropine or hyoscine is substituted, it is likely that the patient will also be sensitive to these drugs which have similar chemical structures. If cyclopentolate, which bears little chemical resemblance to atropine, is substituted there is less chance of cross-hypersensitivity.

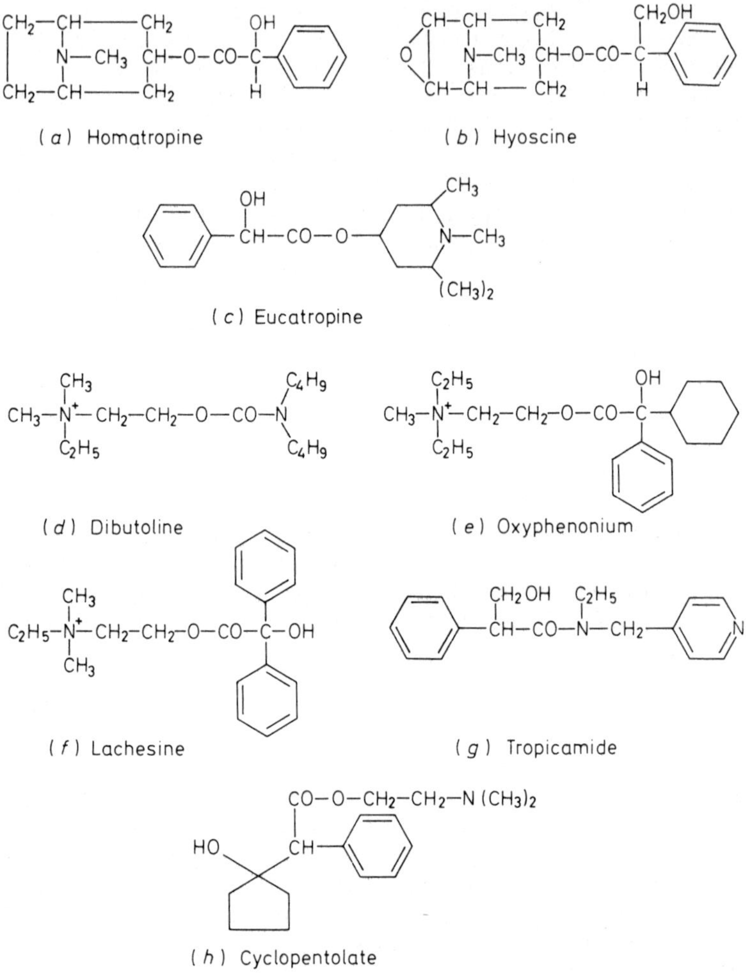

(*a*) Homatropine

(*b*) Hyoscine

(*c*) Eucatropine

(*d*) Dibutoline

(*e*) Oxyphenonium

(*f*) Lachesine

(*g*) Tropicamide

(*h*) Cyclopentolate

Figure 3.2 – The structure of some muscarinic antagonists

After withdrawing the atropine the optician may refer the patient to a general practitioner for treatment. The patient should be assured that this is a temporary condition which will clear quickly. He should also be informed that this condition will recur if he is exposed to atropine-like compounds in the future. The doctor may provide some relief by the sparing use of adrenaline 1:1000, dropped in the conjunctival sac and applied to the skin, zinc ointment may also be applied to the skin. An antihistamine, which antagonizes most of the actions of histamine, may be prescribed; however, as histamine alone is not responsible for all the symptoms and signs of the allergic response some of these may persist despite the antihistamine.

PREPARATIONS

The alkaloid atropine is almost insoluble in water, preparations therefore contain a salt of atropine, generally the sulphate. There are two official preparations of atropine sulphate.

Eye Drops of Atropine Sulphate, BPC, 1973

Atropine sulphate	up to 2 per cent
Phenylmercuric nitrate or sulphate	0.002 per cent
or	
Benzalkonium chloride	0.02 per cent
Purified water	to 100 per cent

The maximum recommended concentration is 2 per cent but a refractionist may prefer to use lower concentrations, for example, 1 per cent. The drops are usually supplied in 10 ml quantities. There is also available single-dose disposable containers of 1 or 2 per cent atropine sulphate solution.

Eye Ointment of Atropine Sulphate, BP, 1973

Atropine sulphate	0.25 or 1.0 per cent
Eye Ointment Basis, BP,	to 100 per cent

The ointment, which is the preferred form, is usually supplied in tubes containing 3 g.

The maximum recommended oral dose of atropine sulphate is 2 mg. A 10 ml bottle of 1 per cent eye drops contains 100 mg of atropine sulphate. A 3 g tube of 1 per cent eye ointment contains 30 mg.

PRACTICAL ASPECTS

The preparations containing atropine are usually restricted to use in young children. The opticians first task is to decide whether or not a cycloplegic is necessary and therefore carry out a pre-cycloplegic examination. Children selected for refraction under atropine will be those with a high amplitude of accommodation who are not reliable in subjective tests. Atropine may also be used in young children with convergent squint to reveal in full the associated refractive error (usually hyperopia). Other indications for atropine use include high esophoria, where there is a need for the fullest possible correction, and pseudomyopia, in order to reveal the true refractive condition.

Atropine may also be used by the ophthalmologist in certain traumatic conditions and to prevent the development of synechiae in inflammatory states.

There are a number of disadvantages associated with the use of atropine preparations which are listed below:

(1) The full cycloplegic effect of atropine is reached only slowly.
(2) Full dilatation of the pupil may make spherical aberration more noticeable in retinoscopy.
(3) The complete cycloplegia necessitates an allowance for tonus.
(4) Cycloplegia is long lasting.
(5) Mydriasis and the loss of the light reflex may result in discomfort.
(6) Atropine is a strong poison.
(7) Atropine can induce allergic responses.

Atropine may precipitate rises in intra-ocular pressure in susceptible people, usually the middle-aged or elderly. In this group there is no need for a potent cycloplegic for refraction.

Homatropine

This is a synthetic compound prepared from mandelic acid and atropine, that is, the tropic acid of atropine is replaced by mandelic acid. Homatropine competes with acetylcholine for the receptor sites on smooth muscle. However, homatropine is less potent than atropine and has a shorter duration of action.

ACTIONS IN THE EYE

Sphincter pupillae

Using drops containing 2 per cent homatropine hydrobromide mydriasis commences in 10–15 minutes and a maximum effect may be reached in less than 30 minutes, although the pupil may not be as fully dilated as with atropine. During the maximum effect the response to light is abolished. With the 2 per cent solution mydriasis may remain maximal for a day, and two days may be needed for full recovery. If lower strengths are used the pupil may return to normal within 24 hours.

Ciliary muscle

After the instillation of 2 per cent drops the amplitude begins to fall in about 15 minutes and proceeds rapidly to a maximum effect in 45–90 minutes. Cycloplegia is not usually as complete as with atropine. Recovery time depends on the dosage employed, but even with the higher concentrations many patients can resume close work in 5–6 hours.

Intra-ocular pressure

Because homatropine has the same mechanism of action as atropine it will produce the same effects on intra-ocular circulation, the iris and canal of Schlemm favouring an increase in intra-ocular pressure. Therefore, homatropine will suffer the same limitations in use as atropine but as homatropine has a shorter duration of action the risk is reduced.

OTHER ACTIONS OF HOMATROPINE

Homatropine inhibits the action of acetylcholine after it is released from postganglionic cholinergic nerves. Thus, it produces the same pharmacological effects as atropine. Unlike atropine it is rarely used systemically but is reserved for ophthalmic use.

PREPARATIONS

Because the alkaloid is almost insoluble in water the hydrobromide salt is used in preparations. The official preparation is:

Eye Drops of Homatropine, BPC, 1973

Homatropine hydrobromide	up to 2 per cent
Benzalkonium chloride	0.02 per cent
or	
Chlorhexidine acetate	0.01 per cent

Purified water to 100 per cent

The usual quantity supplied is 10 ml.

There are also available single-dose disposable units containing a 1 or 2 per cent solution of homatropine hydrobromide. The maximum recommended oral dose of homatropine hydrobromide is 2 mg. A 10 ml bottle of 2 per cent eye drops contains 200 mg.

PRACTICAL ASPECTS

Homatropine is weaker than atropine and cannot produce a complete cycloplegia. It is therefore useful in young adults where complete cycloplegia is not necessary and a shorter recovery time is advantageous. The cases in which homatropine finds most use are those in which a quietening of accommodation allows the true refractive state to be determined, for example, in young people who have restless and spasmodic accommodation, in those patients where the optician suspects a latent error, and in pseudomyopia where it is necessary to break down the spasm to reveal the true error.

The disadvantages of homatropine are essentially those of atropine with the exception that there is a short duration of action and it is not necessary to make an allowance for tonus as cycloplegia is less complete. Caution must be exercised if homatropine is used in elderly patients.

Cyclopentolate

Many atropine-like substances have been synthesized in an attempt to produce compounds active in peptic ulcer. Some were tested in the hope of finding a more ideal cycloplegic, that is, a potent drug with a rapid onset and a short duration of action lacking the toxic potential of atropine. Many were inefficient, painful on instillation or too efficient, having a more prolonged action than atropine. All these were discarded.

Amongst a few compounds having a short-lived, intense action was cyclopentolate, which has sufficient structural similarity to atropine to make it an effective acetylcholine antagonist. However, the difference between the two structures is such that cross-sensitization between the two drugs does not occur. Cyclopentolate can produce a hypersensitivity reaction of itself but the incidence of this phenomenon is less than with atropine.

ACTION IN THE EYE

Mydriasis usually commences in a few minutes and the pupil is widely dilated in about 30 minutes.

The onset of cycloplegia occurs at the same time. The fall in amplitude proceeds rapidly, and even in children it is reduced to 1D or 2D in about 20 minutes. The average time to maximum effect is 30 minutes although it may be as much as 60 minutes in some patients. The average duration of the maximum effect is 45 minutes. Recovery from mydriasis and cycloplegia is quite rapid, the normal amplitude may be regained in 24 hours, recovery of original pupil size taking a little longer.

Cyclopentolate is used as the water-soluble hydrochloride salt. The official preparation is:

Eye Drops of Cyclopentolate, BPC, 1973

Cyclopentolate HCl	up to 1 per cent w/v
Benzalkonium Cl	0.02 per cent w/v
Purified water	to 100 per cent

The drops may also contain boric acid and KCl.

The drops should be stored in a cool place. There are also available single-dose disposable packs containing cyclopentolate HCl, 0.5 and 1.0 per cent.

As cyclopentolate is not used systemically there is no maximum recommended dose quoted.

PRACTICAL ASPECTS

Cyclopentolate may be useful in many of the situations previously discussed under atropine and homatropine. For comparable degrees of cycloplegia it has a shorter recovery period than homatropine and it is not necessary to make an allowance for tonus as the cycloplegia is not complete. A short period of maximum cycloplegia may be regarded by some as a disadvantage because it reduces the time available for the examination. In cases of atropine allergy the optician could choose either homatropine or cyclopentolate as an alternative cycloplegic. Cyclopentolate may be preferred for two reasons. First, the residual accommodation after cyclopentolate is usually less than that found after homatropine. Secondly, homatropine is a close chemical analogue of atropine whereas cyclopentolate has a markedly different structure. Therefore the patient allergic to atropine is likely to be also allergic to homatropine.

There have been no reports of local toxic effects associated with cyclopentolate, however, there are now a number of reports of systemic effects after topical application. These effects are due to an action on the central nervous system causing hallucinations (mainly visual), ataxia, incoherent speech and disorientation. Recovery takes place in some hours with no apparent lasting effects.

As with all cycloplegics there is some danger of inducing raised intra-ocular pressure in susceptible patients.

OTHER CYCLOPLEGICS

Hyoscine

Hyoscine is an alkaloid occurring naturally in certain Solanaceous plants. It is used as the hydrobromide salt.

ACTIONS

The actions of hyoscine are similar to those of atropine at the periphery, it blocks the access of acetylcholine to the muscarinic receptors. Centrally it is a depressant; there is no initial stimulation as seen with atropine.

ACTIONS IN THE EYE

The effects of hyoscine are similar to those of atropine except that it has a much shorter duration of action. Using an 0.5 per cent solution the maximum cycloplegic effect occurs within 40 minutes. The amplitude of accommodation has returned to about 4D in 3–4 hours but full restoration may take more than 24 hours. The effect of hyoscine on the sphincter pupillae slightly preceeds that on the ciliary muscle and lasts slightly longer.

PREPARATIONS

Eye Drops of Hyoscine, BPC, 1973

Hyoscine HBr.	up to 0.5 per cent
Benzalkonium Cl	0.02 per cent
or	
Chlorhexidine acetate	0.01 per cent
Purified water	to 100 per cent

There are also available single-dose disposable packs containing 0.2 per cent hyoscine hydrobromide solution.

Eye Ointment of Hyoscine, BP, 1968

Hyoscine HBr	0.25 per cent
Eye ointment base	to 100 per cent

The maximum recommended oral dose of hyoscine hydrobromide is 0.6 mg. A 10 ml bottle of 0.5 per cent drops contains 50 mg. A 3 g tube of 0.25 per cent ointment contains 7.5 mg.

PRACTICAL ASPECTS

Although more rapid in onset of action than atropine, some variability in the depth of cycloplegia produced in young children has been claimed. However, it has been reported that 2 drops of 0.05 per cent hyoscine can give satisfactory cycloplegia in 1 hour which persists for 6 hours. The child is able to read within 24 hours. Being more potent than atropine there is an increased risk of toxic effects, therefore the value of hyoscine as an atropine substitute is doubtful.

SYNTHETIC ANALOGUES OF ATROPINE

The following four drugs are synthetic analogues of atropine. They are all muscarinic blocking agents and therefore show similar effects to atropine. Dibutoline, oxyphenonium and lachesine do not show the central effects of atropine.

Dibutoline

Dibutoline acts as a cycloplegic and mydriatic by the same mechanism as atropine, that is, competitive inhibition of acetylcholine at muscarinic receptors in the sphincter pupillae and the ciliary muscle. Mydriasis and cycloplegia both have a rapid onset. Using a 5 per cent solution the effects are maximal within 60 minutes and recovery takes 6–12 hours. It is interesting that mydriasis and cycloplegia apparently follow the same time course. It can therefore be assumed that when mydriasis is complete, cycloplegia is also complete (*cf* atropine and most other cycloplegics). Because of its chemical structure the compound has the properties of a wetting agent. The resultant effect is an increase in the rate of penetration, thus providing an explanation for the coincidence of the cycloplegic and mydriatic effects.

Oxyphenonium

This is a potent, long-acting compound prepared as the methylbromide which is water soluble. A 1 per cent solution has similar mydriatic and cycloplegic actions to 1 per cent atropine. It has been particularly recommended where complete cycloplegia is required. Cross-sensitization is unlikely to occur because of the difference in structure.

Lachesine

After instillation of 2 drops of a 1 per cent solution the maximum mydriatic effect is reached in about 1 hour and lasts 5–6 hours. It is a less potent cycloplegic than atropine. The official preparation is:

Eye Drops of Lachesine, BPC, 1973

Lachesine chloride	up to 1 per cent
Phenyl mercuric nitrate/acetate	0.002 per cent
Purified water	to 100 per cent

This drug may be used in patients with atropine allergy.

Tropicamide

This compound is of interest because its mydriatic action is reputed to be more marked than its cycloplegic action. Using a 0.5 or 1 per cent solution mydriasis is rapid in onset, reaching maximum in 15–30 minutes. The pupil is widely dilated. A return to normal occurs within 8–9 hours. Tropicamide has a relatively weak cycloplegic action. The maximum effect is reached after about 25 minutes and is transient. Full amplitude of accommodation has returned at 6 hours. It may be necessary to use repeated instillations to obtain adequate depth and duration of action for refraction.

4

Mydriatics

Mydriatics are used by the refractionist to dilate the pupil for a more complete examination of the fundus, the vitreous and the periphery of the lens, preferably without accompanying cycloplegia. They are more frequently required in elderly patients because: (1) the pupil size decreases with age, and (2) lenticular opacities are more common.

Mydriatics may be useful in young patients when congenital or developmental cataracts prevent a clear view of the fundus or when it is necessary to dilate the pupil to determine the extent and nature of a cataract.

A dilated pupil is essential to examine a fundus thoroughly, and a dilated pupil with abolition of the light reflex is necessary for indirect ophthalmoscopy and slit lamp fundoscopy.

There are two mechanisms by which drugs may produce mydriasis.

(1) Blockade of normal sphincter tone by inhibiting the action of acetylcholine liberated from postganglionic parasympathetic nerves (the muscarinic blocking drugs). Drugs of this type (that is, atropine-like) usually also affect the ciliary muscle which receives the same type of innervation. In order to obtain a selective mydriasis, therefore, it is necessary to choose drugs of low potency relative to atropine or to use lower concentrations of the cycloplegic drugs.

(2) Stimulation of the dilator pupillae will cause a selective mydriasis. Drugs which act in this way mimic the action of noradrenaline liberated from postganglionic sympathetic nerves, and are therefore known as sympathomimetic drugs. Sympathomimetic drugs have little or no effect on the ciliary muscle and therefore may be used without the attendant

complication of cycloplegia. In the eye these drugs will act on the α receptors of smooth muscle (that is, peripheral blood vessels and the dilator pupillae).

Precautions with mydriatics

Mydriasis, with or without accompanying cycloplegia, is more frequently required in elderly patients. Predisposition to glaucoma, and therefore the possibility of a rise in intra-ocular pressure due to blockage of the angle by the iris, is considerably increased in this group of patients. Thus, if mydriasis is required, it is desirable to carry out prior investigations in an attempt to determine whether or not the patient is predisposed. Such investigations might include taking a careful history of the patient, examining the anterior chamber depth and the angle, plotting the fields of vision and measuring the intra-ocular pressure.

If, after the use of a mydriatic, there is some anxiety about a patient then a miotic may be instilled (*see* Chapter 5).

THE MUSCARINIC BLOCKING DRUGS

Because of their action at the sphincter, which is a more powerful muscle than the dilator, their mydriatic effect will be relatively difficult to overcome and the pupillary response to light will be abolished.

Eucatropine

Eucatropine is a synthetic compound having some structural resemblance to atropine (*see Figure 3.2*). Strengths usually employed to produce mydriasis are 2, 5 and 10 per cent. In these concentrations there are no irritant effects on the cornea. Eucatropine has a rapid onset of mydriatic action which develops in 10 minutes and is maximal in about 30 minutes. The mydriatic action has usually disappeared between 6 and 12 hours after instillation. It is unusual to observe any marked effect on accommodation with solutions giving adequate mydriasis.

Homatropine

Most of the relevant information regarding homatropine can be found in the section on cycloplegic drugs. As a mydriatic it is normally used in solutions containing 0.25–0.5 per cent of the hydrobromide salt. With these concentrations mydriasis commences in 10–20 minutes and the pupil is widely dilated in 30 minutes. At this time the pupil is inactive to the stimulus of light. Accommodation is not markedly affected and recovery from the mydriasis commences in 5–10 hours.

Atropine methylbromide and methonitrate

These quaternary derivatives of atropine are fully ionized at the pH of tear fluid and therefore are relatively poorly absorbed. A 1 per cent solution is required for mydriasis which is maximal between 30 minutes and 1 hour, and recovery takes up to 24 hours. For adequate cycloplegia 5 per cent solutions are required, and more than one instillation may be necessary. Even then the cycloplegia is not so complete as with atropine.

Cyclopentolate

Most of the relevant information regarding cyclopentolate can be found in the section on cycloplegic drugs. A concentration of 0.1 per cent has been recommended for use as a mydriatic when cycloplegia is undesirable.

Tropicamide

It has been suggested that tropicamide gives good mydriasis with relatively little disturbance of accommodation. If any such disturbance does occur it is short lived.

THE SYMPATHOMIMETIC DRUGS

The dilator pupillae is less powerful than the sphincter muscle and therefore the mydriasis is not usually as complete as with the muscarinic blocking drugs. The pupillary reflex to light is slowed and incomplete. The effects of these drugs may be reliably reversed with miotics (*see* Chapter 5).

Adrenaline

Adrenaline is a pale buff or white powder, sparingly soluble in water but readily soluble in dilute acid. It is ineffective by the oral route because it is destroyed by alkaline digestive juices. Adrenaline is the natural hormone of the adrenal medulla and chemically is closely related to the sympathetic neurotransmitter noradrenaline. The chemical structure of the sympathomimetic drugs is shown in *Figure 4.1*.

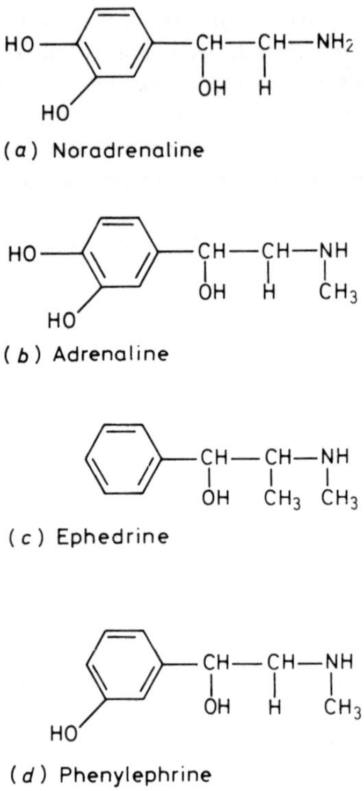

(*a*) Noradrenaline

(*b*) Adrenaline

(*c*) Ephedrine

(*d*) Phenylephrine

Figure 4.1 – The structure of some sympathomimetics

Adrenaline does not dilate the pupil when dropped into the conjunctival sac in the concentration of 0.1 per cent which is the concentration most likely to be used by the ophthalmic optician. If a mydriasis is observed with this concentration then a case of sympathetic hyperirritability is indicated, for example, hyperthyroidism. A pupillary dilatation may occur if the cornea is damaged. A 1 or 2 per cent buffered solution of adrenaline may be used in the treatment of open-angle glaucoma. Mydriasis may accompany the use of these higher concentrations.

Ephedrine

Ephedrine is used as the hydrochloride which is a white crystalline powder. It is water-soluble and a 3.2 per cent solution is isotonic with plasma. It is available as a 5 per cent solution in sterile single-dose disposable packs. Its pharmacological effects are similar to those of adrenaline but the actions are more prolonged and it may be administered orally.

MODE OF ACTION

Because of the structural similarity to adrenaline it was at first suggested that ephedrine acted directly on the same receptors. However, as its effects were reduced by denervation it was suggested that ephedrine acted by inhibiting the breakdown of noradrenaline released from sympathetic nerves. At this time the enzyme monoamine oxidase (MAO) was thought to be the agent responsible for the deactivation of noradrenaline. It is now known that neuronally released noradrenaline is not inactivated by MAO but by uptake into the nerve and the subsequent storage in an inert complex. Therefore an action on MAO does not explain the sympathomimetic effects of ephedrine. It has been demonstrated that ephedrine has a two-fold action at sympathetically innervated tissue. First, it acts directly on the receptor (α or β), an action constituting about 20 per cent of the final response. The remaining 80 per cent of the response is an indirect effect due to an uptake of ephedrine into sympathetic nerves and release of the stored noradrenaline from these nerves, the released noradrenaline then acts on the closely associated receptor.

Action in the eye

A 5 per cent solution of ephedrine hydrochloride begins to dilate the pupil in 5–10 minutes after instillation. The mydriasis is usually sufficient for fundus examination within 20–25 minutes. The maximum mydriatic effect may take longer than 30 minutes.

Some patients may prove resistant to the actions of ephedrine. In older patients with arteriosclerosis the radial blood vessels of the iris have become hardened and will be resistant to the pull of the relatively weak dilator muscle. In these cases one of the muscarinic blocking agents may be required or a mixture of the two types of mydriatic may be preferred. Some resistance to ephedrine may also be seen in patients with heavily pigmented irides.

Although there is no good evidence for the involvement of the sympathetic system in the control of accommodation it has been reported that ephedrine causes some reduction in the amplitude of accommodation within the range 0.5–2 dioptres.

A 5 per cent solution of ephedrine hydrochloride may be used in anisocoria (unequal pupil size) to determine whether the situation is pathological or physiological.

Young patients show no significant change in intra-ocular pressure, there may be some tendency to a slight reduction. A similar effect is seen in older patients with normal anterior chambers but if the angle is narrow and the anterior chamber shallow there is some possibility of a rise.

Phenylephrine

Phenylephrine is closely related in structure to adrenaline (*Figure 4.1*) and is a potent stimulator of the α adrenoceptor with little effect on the β receptor. Unlike ephedrine there is no indirect component of the action of phenylephrine.

It is used as the hydrochloride in solution for 0.5–10 per cent. A 3 per cent solution is isotonic with plasma. The official preparation is:

Phenylephrine Eye Drops, BPC, 1973

Phenylephrine hydrochloride	10 per cent
Sodium citrate	0.3 per cent
Sodium metabisulphite	0.5 per cent
Benzalkonium chloride	0.02 per cent
Purified water to	100 per cent

There are also available single-dose disposable units of a 10 per cent solution.

Action in the eye

When instilled as a 10 per cent solution phenylephrine causes a mydriasis which is maximal in 30–60 minutes. Even a concentration of

0.125 per cent may cause mydriasis, particularly if the cornea is damaged. The effect is of relatively short duration and may be less marked in patients with heavily pigmented irides. There is little effect on accommodation. A fall in intra-ocular pressure may be observed although in elderly patients there is the danger of occluding narrow angles and initiating a rise.

Phenylephrine and other sympathomimetic mydriatics have been observed to release pigment granules from the iris neuroepithelium. It has been suggested that the pigment is released from degenerating cells of the neuroepithelium which rupture during sympathomimetic-induced contraction. This is most prevalent in elderly people and angiosclerosis may constitute a predisposition to this action.

Cocaine

Cocaine is dealt with in detail in the section on local anaesthetics. However, in addition to its local anaesthetic actions cocaine is a mydriatic and vasoconstrictor drug. This is a property peculiar to cocaine and not shared by the other local anaesthetics. Because of its addictive liability cocaine is controlled and not available to the ophthalmic optician.

MODE OF ACTION

Cocaine is an indirectly acting sympathomimetic agent. It inhibits the active uptake of noradrenaline into postganglionic sympathetic nerves. Thus, noradrenaline released from the nerves remains in the synaptic region and reaches concentrations sufficient to activate the α receptors of the smooth muscle of the iris or peripheral blood vessels. There is no direct component of action.

Action in the eye

After instillation of a 2 per cent solution of cocaine mydriasis commences in 5–20 minutes and recovery may take longer than 6 hours. There is little effect on accommodation. The light reflex is still present but reduced. Because of its systemic toxicity and its addictive liability cocaine is not used as a mydriatic agent by the ophthalmic optician although the ophthalmologist may find cocaine of value, for example, in combination with homatropine.

Amphetamine and hydroxyamphetamine

These drugs are indirectly acting sympathomimetics. Their mode of action is similar to ephedrine. Solutions of 1 per cent give mydriasis with no effect on accommodation. However, they have no advantages over ephedrine and phenylephrine. The dangers of amphetamine abuse make it desirable to limit its use as much as possible. Therefore it is not recommended or available for use by the ophthalmic optician.

5

Miotics

Stimulation of the parasympathetic nerve supply to the iris causes release of acetylcholine and contraction of the sphincter pupillae muscle (miosis). Acetylcholine itself is ineffective as a miotic when instilled into the eye as it is rapidly broken down by the enzyme acetylcholinesterase. Thus, other drugs must be used to produce miosis.

There are two types of miotics in use: (1) direct acting miotics which act like acetylcholine but are stable and resistant to cholinesterases (*Figure 5.1*); and (2) the anticholinesterases (*Figure 5.2*).

DIRECT ACTING MIOTICS

These are of two types: (*a*) the cholinomimetic alkaloids; and (*b*) the choline esters.

Pilocarpine

Pilocarpine is a cholinomimetic alkaloid obtained from the leaves of a South American shrub, *Pilocarpus jaborandi.* The base is a colourless liquid of syrupy consistency soluble in water. The official salt is the hydrochloride. (Other cholinomimetic alkaloids are muscarine and arecoline but these are not available for ophthalmic use.)

Pilocarpine has the muscarinic actions of acetylcholine because it is able to occupy the muscarinic receptors present at the junction of post-ganglionic parasympathetic nerves and their effector organs. It is resistant to the hydrolytic action of the cholinesterase enzymes and thus

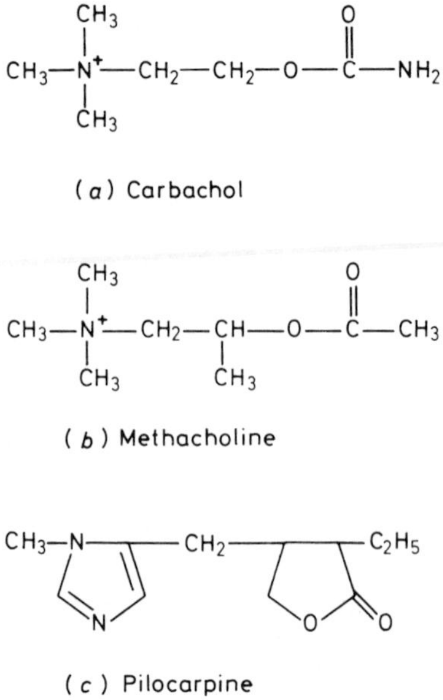

$$(CH_3)_3N^+{-}CH_2{-}CH_2{-}O{-}C(=O){-}NH_2$$

(*a*) Carbachol

$$(CH_3)_3N^+{-}CH_2{-}CH(CH_3){-}O{-}C(=O){-}CH_3$$

(*b*) Methacholine

CH_3—N— —CH_2— —C_2H_5

(*c*) Pilocarpine

Figure 5.1 – The structure of some direct acting miotics

has a useful duration of action. It has relatively little activity at the nicotinic receptors of the ganglia and skeletal muscle. If pilocarpine enters the systemic circulation by absorption from the conjunctival or nasal mucous membranes then the effects seen will be those of stimulating muscarinic receptors and will include an increase in the secretions of the salivary, lacrimal, gastric and pancreatic glands. There will also be increased sweating, an increase in the tone and motility of the gastrointestinal tract, bronchoconstriction and slowing of the heart. In the unlikely event of overdosage all the above effects will occur together with nausea, vomiting, hypotension, tremor and if not treated, death due to respiratory collapse.

ACTIONS IN THE EYE

Sphincter pupillae

With the 1 per cent solution miosis commences in a few minutes and remains marked for about 6 hours. Once the drug has diffused away the

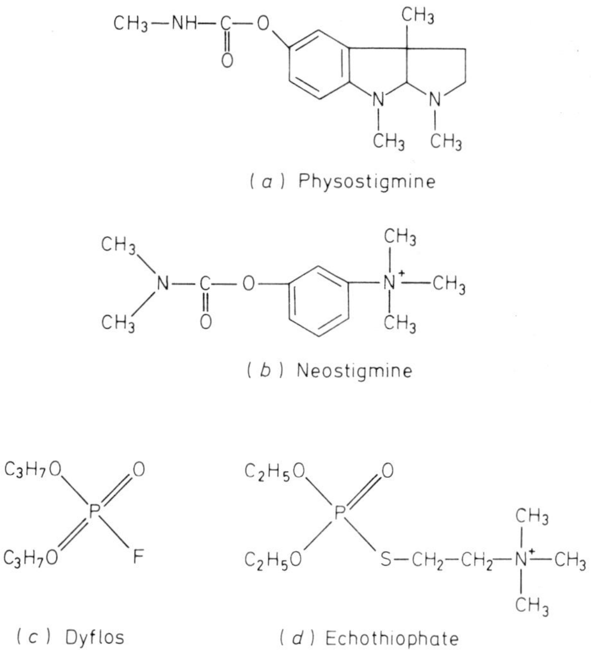

(*a*) Physostigmine

(*b*) Neostigmine

(*c*) Dyflos

(*d*) Echothiophate

Figure 5.2 – The structure of some anticholinesterase miotics

pupil may become larger than normal due to a diminished response of the sphincter to reflex stimulation.

Ciliary muscle

The spasm of accommodation lasts about 1 hour and once recovery begins attempts at close work do not cause the spasm to return. This is an advantage over physostigmine (*see* below).

After instillation pilocarpine causes dilatation of the conjuctival vessels which usually disappears in 30 minutes. Toxic effects after instillations of 1 or 2 drops are uncommon but an allergy may occur if the use is prolonged, as in glaucoma.

PREPARATIONS

Eye Drops of Pilocarpine, BPC, 1973

Pilocarpine hydrochloride	up to 5 per cent

Benzalkonium chloride	0.02 per cent
Purified water	to 100 per cent

Pilocarpine is also available as a 1, 2, 3 and 4 per cent solution of pilocarpine nitrate in single-dose disposable containers.

The maximum recommended oral dose is 12 mg. A 10 ml bottle of 5 per cent eye drops contains 500 mg of pilocarpine hydrochloride.

The choline esters are a group of compounds derived from choline and having similar structures to acetylcholine. They differ from acetylcholine in being more stable and less susceptible to the cholinesterase enzymes. They act directly at the muscarinic receptor and therefore their actions are qualitatively similar to those of pilocarpine. The choline esters have varying ratios of activity at the muscarinic and nicotinic receptors.

Methacholine

A 10 per cent solution is usually required to produce miosis. Lower concentrations are effective if the corneal epithelium is damaged or if a wetting agent is included in the formulation.

Carbachol

This drug has a high nicotinic component in its action, thus part of its miotic effect may be due to a release of acetylcholine from postganglionic parasympathetic nerves. It will also act directly on the muscarinic receptor. Carbachol is virtually resistant to the cholinesterase enzymes and therefore has a sufficiently long duration of action to be useful. Because carbachol has low lipid solubility at any pH it has poor penetrating powers. The presence of benzalkonium chloride in the formulation improves absorption and enhances the drug action.

In concentrations of 0.5–2 per cent carbachol produces a powerful miosis which lasts 3–8 hours, together with spasm of accommodation which is more severe than with pilocarpine and may cause headache. Instillation of carbachol may produce local vasodilatation. Allergic reactions are uncommon.

There is an official preparation:

Eye Drops of Carbachol, BPC, 1973

Carbachol	up to 3 per cent
Benzalkonium chloride	0.02 per cent
Purified water	to 100 per cent

The maximum recommended oral dose is 4 mg. A 10 ml bottle of 3 per cent eye drops contains 300 mg.

ANTICHOLINESTERASES

Anticholinesterases form complexes with cholinesterase enzymes and thereby prevent hydrolysis of acetylcholine (*Figure 5.3*). They are divided into reversible and irreversible inhibitors.

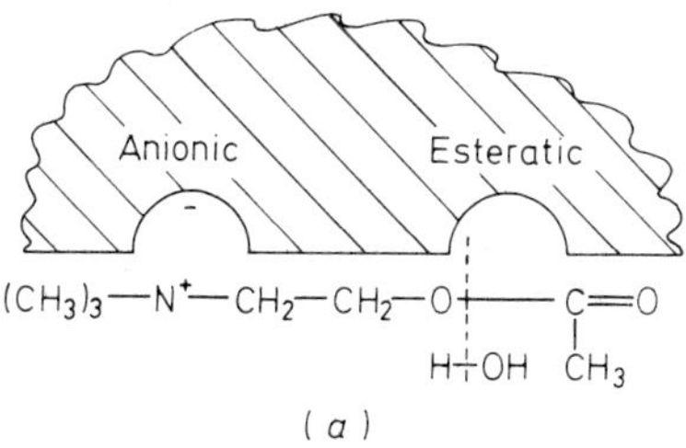

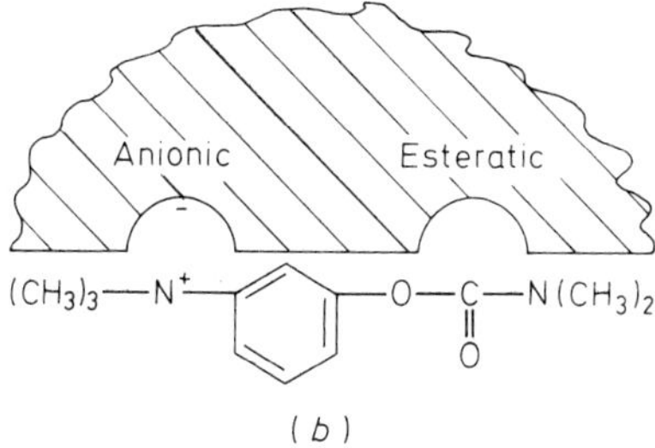

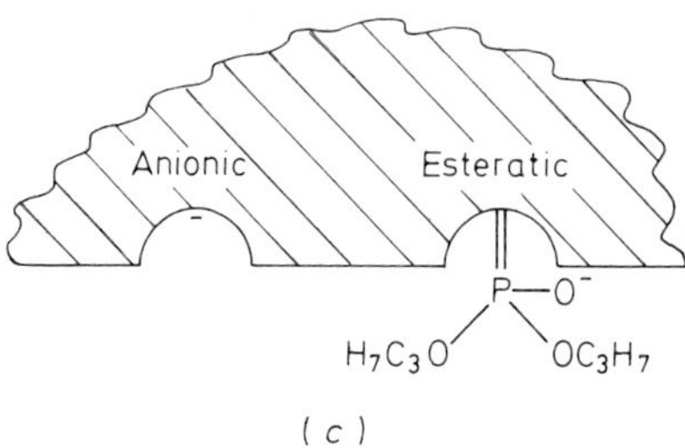

Figure 5.3 – Schematic diagram showing the interaction of acetylcholine, neostigmine and dyflos with acetylcholinesterase. The acetylcholinesterase enzyme has anionic and esteratic sites. (a) Acetylcholine binds to both sites and is rapidly hydrolysed. (b) Neostigmine binds to both sites and is slowly hydrolysed, therefore the enzyme is reversibly blocked. (c) Dyflos phosphorylates the esteratic site, the enzyme is irreversibly blocked

Use of miotics to reverse mydriasis

When a mydriatic drug has been used for fundus examination it may be considered desirable to reverse the mydriasis. This is important if it is suspected that the patient has a predisposition to glaucoma, when a prolonged mydriasis could precipitate a rise in intra-ocular pressure. The miotics generally used are pilocarpine 1 per cent and physostigmine 0.5 per cent or 0.25 per cent. Of these two pilocarpine is probably the agent of choice as there is likely to be less pain.

There are a number of drawbacks to the use of miotics and the indiscriminate reversal of mydriasis is not recommended. Thus, in younger patients the miotic effect and spasm of accommodation may be prolonged and cause more discomfort than would have been experienced with the mydriatic alone. This is most likely to occur if the sympathomimetic group of mydriatics has been used. In other cases when the long-acting cycloplegic drugs (that is, atropine and high concentrations of homatropine) have been used there may be no reversal with either pilocarpine or physostigmine. A more potent miotic is required so that if treatment is desired referral is necessary. If drugs of lower potency are used (cyclopentolate, low concentrations of homatropine) then the result of miotic instillations is variable. In some cases satisfactory reversal may occur. In others the effect of the mydriatic may outlast the effect of the miotic. If there were a predisposition to glaucoma then a second instillation of a miotic would be desirable.

Some of the effects described above are explicable if the differing mechanisms of action of the drugs are understood. The sympathomimetic drugs act on the weak dilator muscle. The miotics act on the stronger sphincter muscle and therefore the mydriasis is relatively easily overcome. It has been suggested that there is pain after the instillation of miotics due to the opposition between the sphincter and dilator muscles. If this is the case then as both pilocarpine and physostigmine act by muscarinic receptor stimulation (pilocarpine directly, physostigmine indirectly) there is no advantage in the use of one or the other in this respect.

The cycloplegic drugs produce mydriasis by a blocking action at the muscarinic receptor on the sphincter muscle. Reversal of this effect relies on a competition between the mydriatic and the miotic agent for these receptors. Drugs with high affinity for the muscarinic receptor, for example, atropine, will be difficult to reverse because it is not possible to achieve a high enough concentration of the miotic agent at the receptor. In the case of pilocarpine the miotic agent is the drug itself. In the case of physostigmine the miotic agent is the accumulated acetylcholine resulting from cholinesterase inhibition. With cyclopentolate and similar drugs the efficiency of reversal is a complex situation depending on the affinity of the cycloplegic and the affinity of the miotic agent for the receptor, the rate of absorption of both types of drugs and their respective time courses of action.

It may occasionally happen that it is desired to use a mydriatic in an elderly patient who has a predisposition to glaucoma. The sympathomimetic drugs used alone may not produce full mydriasis. A combination of ephedrine (5 per cent) and homatropine (0.25 per cent) can be used in this case to give a good mydriasis which is easily reversed because of the low concentration of homatropine. This low concentration is sufficient to cause some block of the sphincter muscle and prevent it opposing the contraction of the dilator muscle. Such combination may also be of use in patients with heavily pigmented irides if mydriasis without cycloplegia is desired.

Reversible anticholinesterases have some similarity in structure to acetylcholine. They combine with the ionic and esteractic sites of the cholinesterase enzyme but are not readily susceptible to hydrolysis.

Physostigmine

This is a naturally occurring compound extracted from the Calabar bean (dried ripe seeds of *Physostigma venenosum*). The pure alkaloid was isolated independently by two groups of people. One group named it physostigmine, the other eserine. These two names are both in common use. The systemic effects of physostigmine are equivalent to excessive stimulation of all cholinergic nerves. Thus, it will potentiate the actions of acetylcholine at the muscarinic receptor and at the nicotinic receptors of ganglia and skeletal muscle. If sufficient physostigmine is absorbed after topical application to the eye, then the symptoms will include salivation, lacrimation, bronchoconstriction, increased tone and motility in the gastro-intestinal tract, increased secretion from mucous glands, possibly nausea and vomiting. slowing of the heart and fasciculation in skeletal muscle followed by muscle weakness. With very high doses effects on the central nervous system occur which include confusion, ataxia, loss of reflexes, convulsions and central respiratory paralysis.

ACTIONS IN THE EYE

Sphincter pupillae

Using a 1 per cent solution of physostigmine sulphate pupillary constriction begins in less than 10 minutes and proceeds rapidly so that the pupil diameter is reduced to less than 2 mm. Marked constriction may persist for more than 12 hours and complete recovery may take a number of days.

Ciliary muscle

The effects of physostigmine on the ciliary muscle begin after the onset of miosis. The ciliary muscle contracts to produce an artificial myopia. The spasm lasts for 2–3 hours. If close work is attempted after this time the spasm may recur. This is because there is sufficient cholinesterase inhibition remaining to cause potentiation of the acetylcholine liberated during the attempt to focus. This feature may remain for several hours.

After instillation physostigmine causes dilatation of the conjunctival vessels accompanied by stinging. The intense spasm of accommodation may result in severe discomfort and the patient often complains of pain over the brow. There may be a twitching of the lids and spasm of the extra-orbital muscles due to potentiation of acetylcholine at the nicotinic receptors. An allergic reaction may develop after prolonged use.

There is an official preparation:

Eye Drops of Physostigmine, BPC, 1973		
Physostigmine sulphate		up to 1 per cent
Sodium metabisulphite		0.2 per cent
Benzalkonium chloride		0.02 per cent
Purified water	to	100 per cent

There is also a combined preparation of physostigmine and pilocarpine:

Eye Drops of Physostigmine and Pilocarpine, BPC, 1973		
Physostigmine sulphate		up to 0.5 per cent
Pilocarpine hydrochloride		up to 4.0 per cent
Sodium metabisulphite		0.2 per cent
Benzalkonium chloride		0.02 per cent
Purified water	to	100 per cent

Physostigmine is relatively unstable and in the absence of the antoxidant sodium metabisulphite rapidly turns pink to deep red, due to the formation of rubreserine. This product of oxidation is also a miotic compound but is irritant. Sodium metabisulphite delays the appearance of the red oxidation product partly by a decolorizing action. Therefore there is a limited storage period for physostigmine which should be observed even if the solution has not discoloured.

Neostigmine

This has a similar mode of action to physostigmine. It is highly ionized in aqueous solution and therefore is relatively poorly absorbed after topical application, and the response may vary from patient to patient. It is stable in solution. No official preparation is available. Proprietary preparations containing neostigmine 3 per cent are manufactured and used mainly in the treatment of glaucoma.

Irreversible or long-acting anticholinesterases have an extremely long duration of action. They are usually organo-phosphorus compounds which act at the esteratic site of the cholinesterase enzyme (*Figure 5.3*). Cholinesterase activity can only be restored by synthesis of new enzyme material which explains their prolonged duration of action. These compounds are potent and extremely toxic and should be used with caution under medical supervision. They include dyflos and echothiophate. The organo-phosphorus compounds are more efficient inhibitors of cholinesterase than acetylcholinesterase, unlike the reversible anticholinesterases which inhibit both types of enzymes equally.

As well as the dangers of systemic effects due to absorption after instillation these substances have two other serious disadvantages, if their use is prolonged. There is the danger of delayed neurotoxicity, nerves become demyelinated and there is a spastic paralysis followed by a flaccid paralysis in skeletal muscle. The second disadvantage is the possibility of long-term use causing lens opacities.

A compound with a long duration of action which is not of the organo-phosphorus type is demecarium. This substance is synthesized from two molecules of neostigmine connected together by a carbon chain. It is water-soluble and stable. This drug will produce a miosis which is maximum in 2–4 hours and is sustained for 5–7 days after instillation of an 0.5 per cent solution. After systemic absorption side-effects are those that would be expected of cholinesterase inhibition.

Dyflos

Dyflos is a colourless oily liquid which is volatile and unstable in water. It may be used in glaucoma as a 0.1 per cent solution in arachis oil. It causes pronounced miosis and ciliary spasm.

Echothiophate

Echothiophate is a compound with a similar type of action to dyflos but is more stable in aqueous solution than dyflos, with a half-life of days rather than hours. It may be prepared in aqueous solution as the iodide salt. Benzalkonium chloride which is incompatible with iodides should not be used as a preservative. There is no official preparation but it is marketed in proprietary preparations containing up to 0.25 per cent.

6

Local Anaesthetics

Local anaesthetics are used to reversibly block pain sensation in relatively restricted areas of the body. When applied in effective concentrations they are able to block nerve conduction in all parts of the nervous system and in all types of nerve fibres (both motor and sensory nerves). They will also block conduction in the heart and other conducting tissues. Sensitivity to touch, pressure, heat and cold is also abolished.

METHODS OF APPLICATION

Topical anaesthesia

The local anaesthetic is applied to a surface as a solution, ointment, cream or powder.

Infiltration anaesthesia

The local anaesthetic is injected by the subcutaneous route in order to affect the fine sensory nerve branches.

Nerve block anaesthesia

The local anaesthetic is injected near to a major nerve trunk. Block of conduction of impulses in motor and sensory nerves results. Therefore there is muscle relaxation as well as loss of sensation.

Spinal anaesthesia

The local anaesthetic is injected into the subarachnoid space producing analgesia and muscle relaxation without the patient losing consciousness.

Properties of an ideal local anaesthetic

(1) Rapid onset of action.
(2) Profound depth of anaesthesia.
(3) Adequate duration for the purpose required.
(4) Reversible action.
(5) No pain at site of administration.
(6) No after pain when the effects wear off.
(7) No hypersensitivity or allergic reactions.
(8) No local or systemic toxicity.
(9) Compatible with any other drug used, including preservatives.
(10) Preferably water-soluble, stable in solution and on autoclaving.

Further requirements for use in the eye

(1) Good penetration.
(2) No irritant or damaging effect on the cornea.
(3) No pupil effect.
(4) No vasodilatation.

Uses in ophthalmic optics

(1) Moulding technique in contact lens fitting.
(2) Tonometry.
(3) Removal of foreign bodies.
(4) Gonioscopy.

There are certain dangers associated with the use of local anaesthetics in the eye. If a patient is allowed to leave the consulting room before recovery from the effects of a local anaesthetic, then damage may unwittingly be caused as the anaesthetized cornea cannot detect the presence of a foreign body. Repeated instillations of local anaesthetics may result in desquamation of the corneal epithelial cells because normal functioning of the nerves is needed for their survival. These effects on the cornea are aggravated by the loss of the protective blink reflex and drying of the eye. This may result in pitting and ulceration of the cornea.

MODE OF ACTION

Before discussing how local anaesthetics produce their effect it is necessary to review the current concepts on how a nerve impulse is generated and transmitted.

A nerve is composed of a bundle of nerve fibres, each nerve fibre (*Figure 6.1*) consisting of the following:

(1) The axon, a core of semi-fluid gelatinous material.

(2) A protein-lipid membrane which surrounds the axon.

(3) In some fibres a myelin sheath which surrounds the membrane. This is interrupted at intervals by the nodes of Ranvier, which are gaps in the myelin sheath.

The inside of the nerve fibre is electrically negative with respect to the outside (*Figure 6.1*). This potential difference is about 50–70 mV and is known as the membrane potential. A potential exists because there is a slight excess of negative ions within the cell and a slight excess of positive ions without (*Figure 6.2*). This situation arises because of the following:

(1) The resting nerve cell membrane exhibits differences in permeability towards various ions, in particular Na^+ and K^+. There is a very low permeability to Na^+ ions.

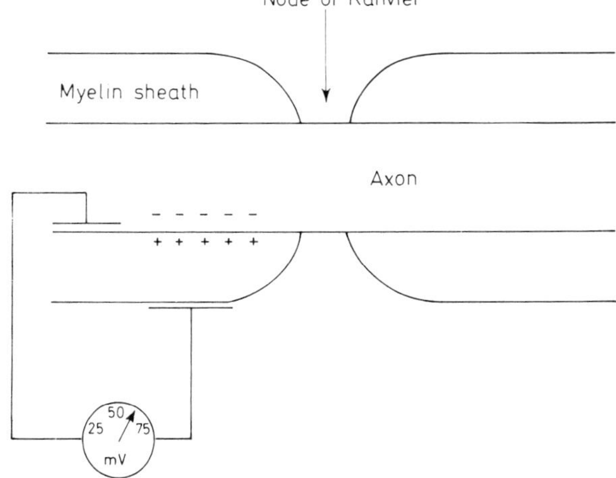

Figure 6.1 – Diagram of a myelinated nerve fibre

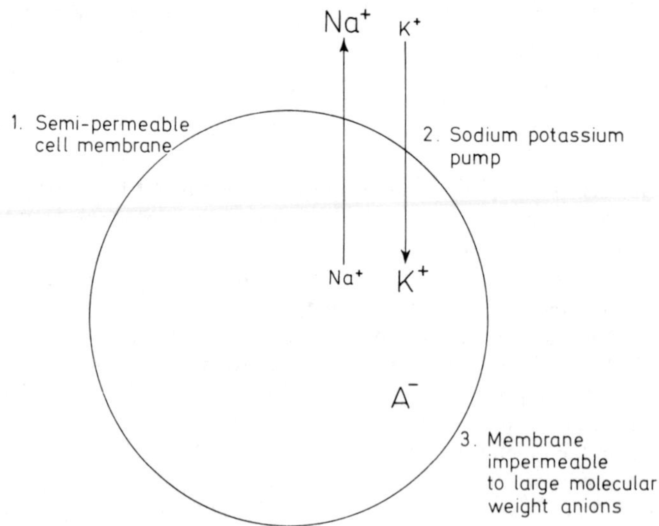

Figure 6.2 – The distribution of anions and cations across a nerve cell membrane

(2) There is a Na^+/K^+ pump in the membrane which keeps Na^+ outside the nerve and brings K^+ ions into the nerve. The pump requires energy from metabolic processes.

(3) The impermeability of the membrane to certain anions, for example, sulphate and phosphate, maintaining them (A^-) within the cell.

If a potential difference were applied between the extracellular fluid and the cytoplasm it would not be transmitted very far along the fibre but for the fact that the fibre exhibits threshold behaviour, that is, electrical instability. The ionic differences responsible for the membrane potential constitute a store of potential energy, and this is made use of in threshold behaviour. If a sub-threshold impulse is applied there is a small depolarization of the cell (inside of the cell becomes less negative) which rapidly dies away (*Figure 6.3*). If the strength of the applied impulse is increased the cell is depolarized to the threshold level and a propagated action potential occurs. This travels the length of the nerve fibre without any decrease in magnitude. The threshold is about 20 mV lower than the resting potential. Once the stimulus is sufficient to depolarize the cell to the threshold increasing it has no effect on the size of the propagated action potential. It can be shown that during the action potential there is a small increase in the Na^+ ion concentration inside the fibre and a small decrease in the K^+ ion concentration. There

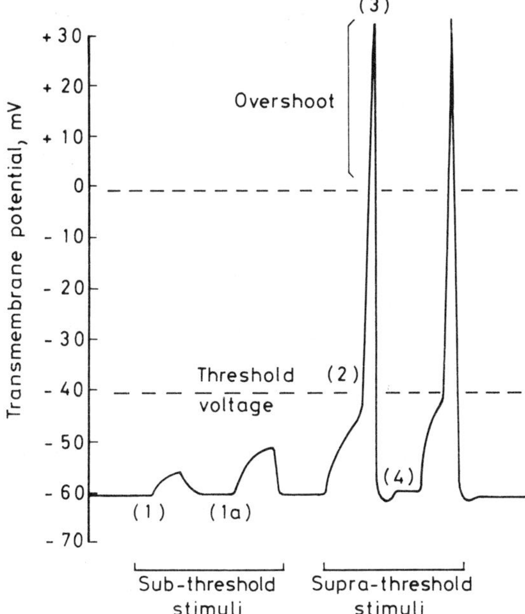

Figure 6.3 – Changes in the transmembrane potential of a nerve fibre due to sub-threshold and supra-threshold stimulation. (1) and (1a) Sub-threshold stimuli. (2) At this point the large increase in the permeability to sodium occurs and the sodium ions enter the nerve fibre causing a reversal of polarity. (3) At this point the increase in permeability to potassium occurs and the potassium ions leave the nerve fibre tending to restore the nerve transmembrane potential. (4) At this point the nerve has returned to its resting state, it is relatively impermeable to sodium and potassium ions and the sodium pump is effective.

is an increase in the membrane permeability to Na^+ and this ion enters during depolarization. At the peak of the action potential, about +30–40 mV, the membrane permeability to Na^+ ions decreases and the permeability to K^+ ions increases. These two factors are responsible for repolarization. In this situation K^+ is lost from the nerve. In fact, the nerve becomes slightly hyperpolarized because the permeability to K^+ ions is still above that found in the resting nerve when the permeability to Na^+ has returned to normal.

Conduction

An action potential is sufficient to supply a supra-threshold stimulus to adjacent regions of the membrane. Local circuit currents are generated, passing from the active to the inactive region within the cell, and from the inactive to the active outside the cell. In this way an action potential is propagated along the nerve fibres. In myelinated nerves the changes in membrane permeability and thus the action potentials occur only at the nodes of Ranvier due to the insulating effect of the myelin at other sites. Thus, the depolarizations pass from node to node. There is therefore an increase in conduction velocity. This type of conduction is called saltatory conduction.

An understanding of how local anaesthetics act comes predominantly from studies on easily accessible, large, myelinated fibres described above. Sensory nerve endings, such as those found in the cornea, are non-myelinated. These nerves have not been so well studied. However, from experiments on the myelinated fibres one can predict how local anaesthetics will affect nerve impulse generation and conduction in fine sensory nerves. In the following discussion it is assumed that the action of local anaesthetics on membranes is the same in both types of nerve.

Local anaesthetics prevent both the generation and conduction of nerve impulses. The site of action is the membrane. Here they prevent the large, transient increase in the permeability to Na^+ ions and also reduce the resting permeability to K^+ ions. The local anaesthetic becomes bound to the outer layers of the membrane but it is not known how this binding stabilizes the permeability of the membrane. One suggestion is that local anaesthetics increase the surface pressure of the lipid layer of the membrane, this could close pores through which the ions move. Such an action would result in a general decrease in resting permeability and limit the increase in membrane permeability to Na^+ ions. This suggestion is based on observations that the anaesthetic potency of a series of compounds parallels their ability to increase the surface pressure of artificial mono-molecular lipoid films.

STRUCTURE AND CHEMISTRY

There is a great deal of similarity in the structure of local anaesthetics. Most local anaesthetics are tertiary amines (that is, ammonia, NH_3, with all three hydrogen atoms replaced by other groups) but a few are secondary amines. They have the general structure: lipophilic portion; linkage; hydrophilic portion (*Figure 6.4*). The structure of individual local anaesthetics is shown in *Figure 6.5*.

The lipophilic portion gives lipid solubility, the hydrophilic portion water solubility. As is discussed in the section on drug absorption a good balance of these two properties is essential for absorption into the

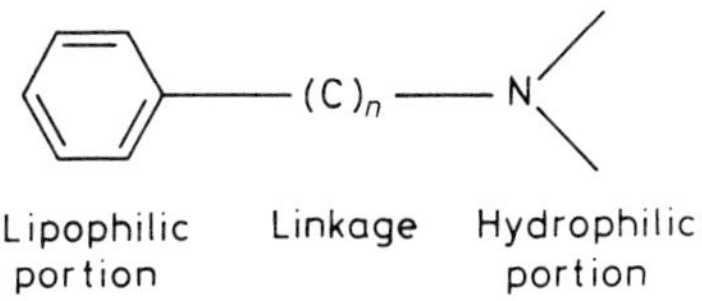

Lipophilic portion — $(C)_n$ — N (Linkage) — Hydrophilic portion

Figure 6.4 – The general structure of local anaesthetics

layers of the cornea. The hydrocarbon chain connecting these two portions contains an ester or amide linkage and maintains correctly the fairly critical distance between the lipophilic and hydrophilic portions. A chain length equivalent to 2 or 3 carbon atoms is the best length for this linkage. The type of linkage can affect metabolism and therefore the duration of action.

The ester link

$$-\overset{\displaystyle O}{\overset{\|}{C}}-O-CH_2-$$

as in procaine is easily hydrolysed by the enzyme cholinesterase (non-specific) of plasma. Therefore, local anaesthetics with unprotected ester linkages have a short duration of action.

The amide link

$$NH-\overset{\displaystyle O}{\overset{\|}{C}}-CH_2-$$

as in lignocaine is much more resistant to hydrolysis and therefore local anaesthetics with this link are likely to be longer acting.

Local anaesthetics are weak bases, relatively insoluble in water and rather unstable. They readily form water-soluble salts of strong acids which are stable in solution. Local anaesthetics are therefore generally supplied as the hydrochloride salt. The unionized form is important for absorption. However, it is the ionized form, the cation, which is responsible for the local anaesthetic effect. (For a more detailed discussion of this aspect *see* Appendix.)

	Lipophilic portion	Linkage	Hydrophilic portion
Cocaine	C_6H_5–C(=O)	–O–CH–CH_2–CH–; CH_2–CH_2; CH($COOCH_3$)	N–CH_3; CH
Procaine	H_2N–C_6H_4–C(=O)	–O–CH_2–CH_2–	N(C_2H_5)(C_2H_5)
Amethocaine	H_9C_4(H)N–C_6H_4–C(=O)	–O–CH_2–CH_2–	N(CH_3)(CH_3)
Oxybuprocaine	H_9C_4O, H_2N–C_6H_3–C(=O)	–O–CH_2–CH_2–	N(C_2H_5)(C_2H_5)
Proxymetacaine	H_7C_3O, H_2N–C_6H_3–C(=O)	–O–CH_2–CH_2–	N(C_2H_5)(C_2H_5)
Lignocaine	CH_3, CH_3–C_6H_3–N(H)	–C(=O)–CH_2–	N(C_2H_5)(C_2H_5)
Butacaine	H_2N–C_6H_4–C(=O)	–O–CH_2–CH_2–CH_2–	N(C_4H_9)(C_4H_9)

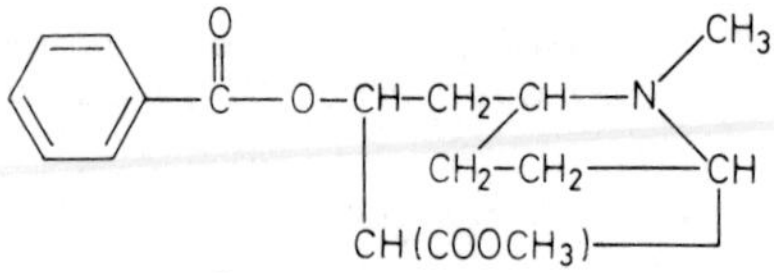

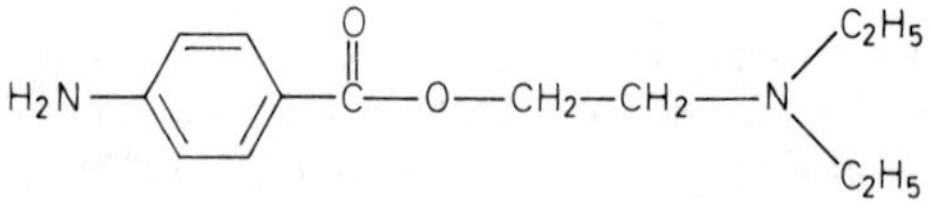

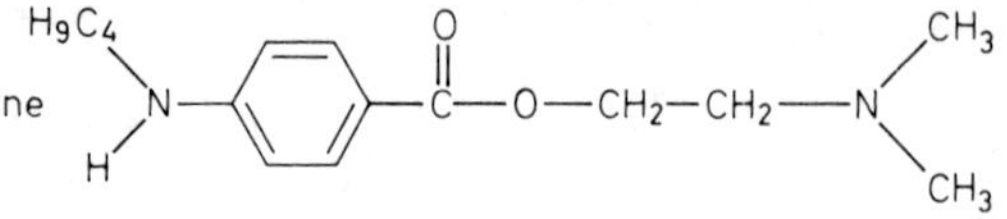

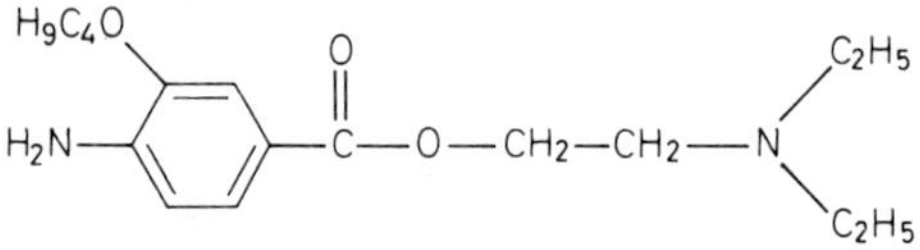

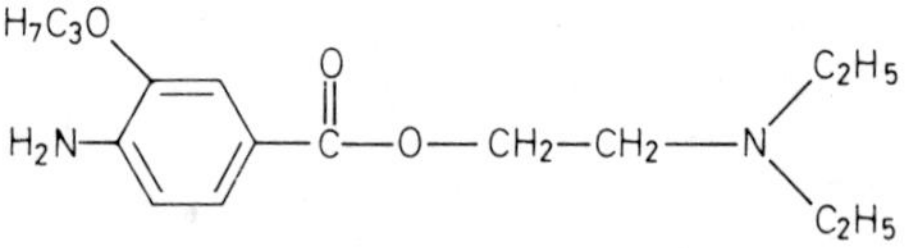

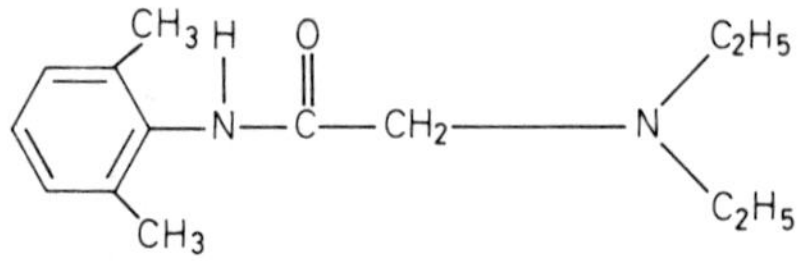

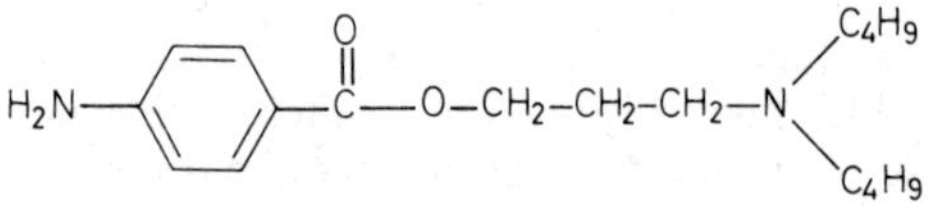

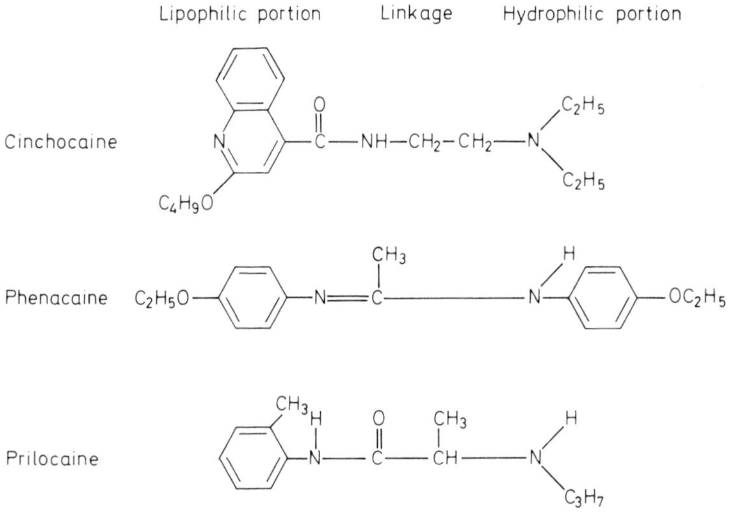

Figure 6.5 – The structure of individual local anaesthetics

ONSET AND DURATION OF ANAESTHESIA

Generally, small nerve fibres are more susceptible to local anaesthetics than are large fibres, and unmyelinated nerve fibres are more susceptible than myelinated fibres, the myelin providing a further barrier to absorption. Susceptibility does not depend on the type of fibre (that is, motor or sensory).

For a given nerve fibre the time to the onset of action depends on the concentration of the local anaesthetic, the diffusion time, the nerve diameter and the pH of the solution used (this last affects ionization and therefore absorption: *see* Appendix). Recovery time depends on the bond between the local anaesthetic and the membrane, the fibre size and the rate of removal of the drug. The rate of removal depends, in turn, on factors such as the vascularity of the area and the ease of hydrolysis of the drug. The higher the blood supply the higher the rate of removal. Some local anaesthetics, for example, procaine, are vasodilators and easily removed from the site, others such as cocaine are vasoconstrictors and are retained at the site.

ABSORPTION, METABOLISM AND EXCRETION

Even after topical application some local anaesthetics will enter the blood. They are removed from the blood by tissue redistribution, metabolic inactivation and excretion. Ester-linked compounds are readily hydrolysed, amide-linked compounds are less easily hydrolysed. Further metabolism takes place in the liver and the metabolites and unchanged drug excreted through the kidneys.

TOXICITY

Allergic reactions to the ester-linked compounds are not uncommon. These reactions may take the form of a dermatitis or asthma. Reactions to the amide-linked compounds are rare.

It is unusual to see systemic toxic effects of local anaesthetics other than cocaine after local application. The advent of systemic toxicity depends on the elevation of the blood levels and the length of time for which they are elevated. Most conspicuous reactions are convulsions (a central nervous system effect) but the most dangerous are respiratory depression and hypotension. Cocaine is unique in causing marked cortical stimulation. Some people are especially sensitive to cocaine and cardiovascular collapse may occur after small doses.

Cocaine

Cocaine is an alkaloid which occurs naturally in the leaves of *Erythroxylon coca*. Its possession is controlled by the law because of its addictive liability. Thus, it is not available to the non-medical optician. However, as it was the first local anaesthetic used it may serve as a standard with which to compare the synthetic local anaesthetics.

It is potent and well absorbed after topical application. It is normally used as 2 per cent drops which give complete anaesthesia in 10–15 minutes. Partial anaesthesia may remain for about an hour. Cocaine may damage the cornea, causing pitting and ulceration. Because it potentiates noradrenaline it causes mydriasis, and vasoconstriction which may be of use in ophthalmic surgery, providing a bloodless field. Potentiation of adrenaline liberated from the adrenal medulla may be the major factor in cocaine's toxic effect on the heart. Because of the danger of corneal damage, toxicity and addiction it is not much used.

It is obvious from the above statements that cocaine does not conform to the properties of an ideal local anaesthetic as listed at the beginning of this Chapter. The slow onset and long duration of action make it desirable that alternatives be available.

Procaine

Procaine was the first of the synthetic local anaesthetics to come into wide use. However, it is of little value for topical application. It is only poorly absorbed and its action is slow to develop. Surgeons may use it by sub-conjunctival injection as a 5–10 per cent solution. When used in infiltration anaesthesia it is given with a vasoconstrictor such as adrenaline to prolong its action. It is hydrolysed to para-aminobenzoic acid and therefore should be avoided in patients receiving sulphonamide treatment (*see* Chapter 8).

Amethocaine

Amethocaine has been widely used by opticians. It is well absorbed; 0.5–1.0 per cent drops give adequate corneal anaesthesia. The blink reflex is absent after 10–15 seconds. The duration is sufficient for moulding, tonometry or foreign-body removal. Local responses to amethocaine are rare but superficial corneal epithelial lesions may occur after prolonged or repeated use. There is some initial stinging after instillation of the drops.

The official formulation of the BPC, 1973, is:

Amethocaine hydrochloride	up to 1 per cent
Sodium metabisulphite	0.1 per cent
Phenyl mercuric nitrate or acetate	0.002 per cent
Purified water	to 100 per cent

It is also available as 0.5 and 1 per cent solution in single-dose disposable containers.

Oxybuprocaine

Oxybuprocaine is well absorbed. A single instillation of 0.3 or 0.4 per cent gives sufficient anaesthesia for tonometry in less than 60 seconds. With a second drop at 90 seconds anaesthesia is sufficient for contact lens work. A third drop after a further 90 seconds gives anaesthesia which is sufficient for foreign-body removal. Full recovery from three drops occurs in one hour. There is no prior irritation, no action on blood vessels or pupil and no evidence of corneal damage. Some proprietary preparations of oxybuprocaine contain chlorhexidine acetate as a preservative. This preservative is incompatible with fluorescein because a dense precipitate forms on mixing.

Oxybuprocaine is available in single-dose disposable packs which contain no preservative.

Proxymetacaine

Proxymetacaine is well absorbed; the onset, depth and duration of anaesthesia are similar to those for oxybuprocaine. Recovery from 1 to 2 drops of a 0.5 per cent solution takes about 15 minutes. No prior irritation occurs and there is no evidence of corneal damage. The drops discolour on exposure to air with an accompanying loss of potency. Drops should be stored in the refrigerator after opening but not allowed to freeze. The preparation should also be protected from light.

Lignocaine

A 2 per cent solution of lignocaine is effective at the cornea, giving a more rapid, more intense, more extensive and more prolonged effect than an equal concentration of procaine. There is no effect on the pupil.

Factors which contribute to the longer duration of local anaesthetic action are the absence of marked vasodilation and a resistance of the compound to hydrolysis. Lignocaine is resistant to hydrolysis because it has an amide rather than an ester link, and because of two methyl substituents on the benzene ring of the lipophilic moiety. The groups prevent the close approach of the drug to the active sites on the cholinesterase enzyme (steric hindrance) thereby inhibiting the hydrolytic action of the enzyme.

Butacaine

Butacaine has a similar potency to cocaine but a more rapid onset and a more prolonged action. One drop of a 2 per cent solution gives sufficient anaesthesia for foreign-body removal. Butacaine has no effect on the pupil or blood vessels and adverse effects on the cornea are rare. It finds more use in ophthalmology than in ophthalmic optics.

Cinchocaine

Cinchocaine is the most potent, most toxic and most long-acting of the local anaesthetics used for topical application. It may be used in 0.1 per cent solutions for corneal anaesthesia (*cf* 2 per cent cocaine). The drops should be protected from light.

Phenacaine

Phenacaine is another local anaesthetic with a potency and toxicity similar to cocaine. A 1 per cent solution is well absorbed and has no effect on the pupil. It causes vasodilatation and smarting.

Prilocaine

Prilocaine is a relatively new local anaesthetic which has twice the potency of procaine. The onset and duration of action are similar to lignocaine. It has not yet been widely used for corneal anaesthesia. There is some possibility of methaemoglobinaemia resulting from its systemic use.

7

Staining Agents

Staining agents are used by the ophthalmic optician to determine the accuracy of fit of hard contact lenses or as diagnostic aids. They may be used to reveal damage to the cornea and conjunctiva or to detect conditions of the epithelial cells which may influence contact lens tolerance.

Fluorescein

Fluorescein as its sodium salt is available in three types of ophthalmic preparation.

Eye drops

Fluorescein Eye Drops, BPC, 1973	
Fluorescein sodium	up to 2 per cent
Phenyl mercuric nitrate	0.002 per cent
Purified water	to 100 per cent

Sterile fluorescein papers

These are prepared from filter paper soaked with a 20 per cent solution. The papers are then packed and autoclaved to provide a sterile disposable unit. If the eye is moist sufficient fluorescein may be released by placing the strip in the conjunctival sac for a few seconds. A method which has been recommended to provide a greater volume of fluorescein solution is to crease the strip longitudinally (before opening the sterile pack) remove the strip and place a drop of sterile water or isotonic saline solution in the crease. The fluorescein solution so prepared can be transferred to the eye.

Sterile single-dose disposable units

These contain 2 per cent fluorescein sodium without a preservative. They may be used to replace the multidose preparations when larger volumes of fluorescein than are provided by the papers are required.

Multidose containers of fluorescein are very liable to bacterial contamination. *Pseudomonas aeruginosa* is among the commoner contaminants. This organism can produce corneal destruction, and it is likely to be resistant to a wide range of antibiotics making the treatment difficult. Many of the common preservatives (benzalkonium chloride and chlorbutol) are inactivated and chlorhexidine acetate is incompatible with fluorescein. Because of this serious disadvantage the disposable sterile units are to be preferred.

MODE OF ACTION

Fluorescein is a water-soluble compound which appears yellow in colour but exhibits a green fluorescence in alkaline conditions. Because of its poor lipid solubility it will not penetrate intact cell membranes. If there is damage to the cells of the epithelial layer then fluorescein gains access to Bowman's membrane, the stroma and even the aqueous. Thus, the stain is taken up by damaged tissue which can be visualized as a green fluorescence in contrast to the yellowish-green appearance of the dye on the undamaged surfaces. If the eye is irrigated with normal saline solution to remove excess fluorescein the damaged areas are more easily visualized. As the tissue regenerates the colour disappears. Fluorescein drops are non-toxic, locally or systemically, and are non-irritant, even in the presence of damaged tissue.

USES

Detection of corneal damage

Fluorescein may be used to demonstrate the integrity of corneal epithelium and damage to the conjunctiva.

Contact lens fitting

Fluorescein can be used to identify faults in the fitting of hard contact lenses; the dimensions of the spaces between the lens and the cornea are determined by the amount of colour present. If viewed with blue light areas of contact between the lens and cornea will be seen as dull purple patches. Any superficial corneal damage during fitting will also be detected. Fluorescein should not be used with soft contact lens as it is absorbed by the lens material.

Detection of foreign bodies

Foreign bodies which are present on the cornea may be more easily detected if fluorescein and a blue light are used. The foreign body is surrounded by a ring of stain which appears green.

Patency of lacrimal ducts

If it is suspected that the naso-lacrimal ducts are blocked fluorescein is a useful diagnostic aid. Fluorescein drops are instilled and if the lacrimal ducts are patent then it may be detected in the nasal and oral secretions.

Applanation tonometry

Fluorescein, 0.06 per cent, may be used in applanation tonometry. Local anaesthetic drops are instilled to anaesthetize the cornea, followed by fluorescein drops.

Fluorescein is also used by ophthalmologists for fundus photography and studies of aqueous flow. An interesting use of fluorescein is in the inactivation of methyl violet, a dye which is used in indelible pencils. Local damage with an indelible pencil may lead to the spreading of the dye through ocular tissues where the toxic effects may produce serious delayed damage. Irrigation with 2 per cent fluorescein will precipitate excess dye which can be washed from the eye.

Rose bengal

This is a brownish-red solid soluble, 1 part in 4 parts water. It is available as a 1 per cent solution in sterile single-dose disposable units.

USES

Rose bengal stains degenerate cells and their nuclei, and may thus be used to locate degenerate tissue in the sclera and conjunctiva. The presence of facial skin conditions (for example, various forms of dermatitis) may indicate that the cornea and conjunctiva are also affected. Rose bengal may help to diagnose whether or not the ocular tissues are involved. Such tissue would be stained a red colour not removed by irrigation with saline solution. Care should be taken if local anaesthetic solutions have been used previously as a false positive may be obtained. There is likely to be more irritation after instillation of rose bengal than fluorescein. Particular care should be taken during instillation to avoid overspill onto lids and facial tissues as the staining is relatively persistent.

The use of rose bengal after the wearing of contact lens will indicate any areas where the lens presses on the cornea and may indicate errors in fitting.

Rose bengal will also stain mucous deposits. In order, therefore, to differentiate between degenerate tissue and mucous a second stain may be required. Alcian blue, 1 per cent, which preferentially stains mucous may be used for this purpose. This stain should not be used if the cornea is deeply eroded because of prolonged discoloration of exposed connective tissue.

8
Antimicrobial Agents

The sulphonamides

These are synthetic compounds which have a structural similarity to para-aminobenzoic acid (PABA).

MODE OF ACTION

Some bacteria require PABA for growth and multiplication. These bacteria use the PABA to synthesize the vitamin folic acid. When a bacterial cell is exposed to sulphonamides the synthesis of folic acid is blocked due to the competition between the sulphonamide and PABA for the enzyme folic acid synthetase. The similarities between PABA and sulphonamides are shown in *Figure 8.1*. Human cells do not synthesize folic acid but obtain their supply by absorption from the gastrointestinal tract. Therefore, human cells are not affected by sulphonamides.

Sulphonamides have a relatively broad spectrum, acting against Gram-positive as well as Gram-negative bacteria. In the concentrations used they are usually bacteriostatic (that is, they inhibit growth and multiplication), in higher concentrations they may be bactericidal.

Preparations for ophthalmic use

Sulphacetamide sodium is the sulphonamide most widely used by the ophthalmic optician although a preparation containing sulphafurazole is

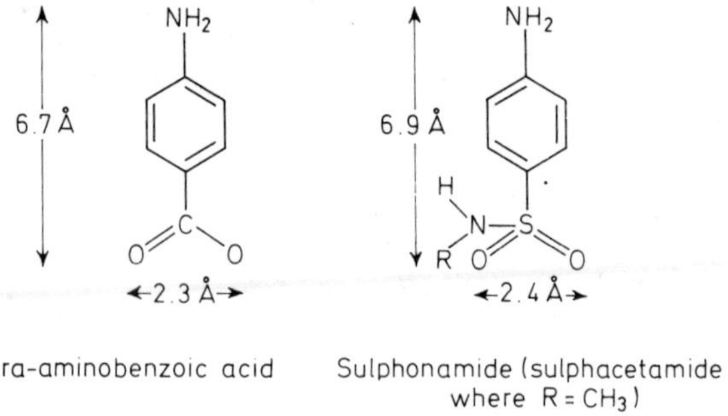

Para-aminobenzoic acid

Sulphonamide (sulphacetamide where $R = CH_3$)

Figure 8.1 – The molecular structure of para-aminobenzoic acid compared with that of sulphonamides

available. Sulphacetamide sodium is soluble in water giving solutions which are less alkaline than the solutions of most other sulphonamides. Sulphacetamide drops are available in concentrations of 10, 20 and 30 per cent in multidose containers, 10 and 30 per cent in single-dose disposable containers. Sulphacetamide eye ointment is available in concentrations of 2.5, 6 and 10 per cent. Sulphafurazole is marketed in drops containing 4 per cent. There is also a preparation containing 10 per cent sulphacetamide and 0.1 per cent zinc sulphate.

USES

Sulphacetamide drops in a concentration of 10 per cent may be used prophylactically after contact lens work, removal of a foreign body or in other situations in which corneal abrasions are likely to have occurred. The value of this practice is questionable because of the short duration of the bacteriostatic action after instillation. Even the 10 per cent drops are hypertonic and may cause stinging. Although drops of a higher concentration are available these are usually reserved for the treatment of corneal, conjunctival and lid infections. The use of these drops would be therapeutic rather than prophylactic. The ointment causes less discomfort than the drops and remains longer in the eye.

Propamidine and dibromopropamidine isethionate

These antibacterial agents are bacteriostatic, bactericidal and also fungistatic. The dibromo compound is available as an eye ointment containing 0.15 per cent. It has a wide range of activity, including an action against Gram-negative bacilli and some strains of *Pseudomonas aeruginosa*. Propamidine is available in isotonic solution at a concentration of 0.1 per cent. It also has a wide range of activity but is not active against *Pseudomonas aeruginosa.*

Antibiotics

The early antibiotics were substances elaborated by microorganisms which possessed either bacteriostatic or bactericidal activity. Many of the present antibiotics are synthetic derivatives of these substances. The sale and supply of antibiotics is controlled by law and these drugs are therefore not generally available to the ophthalmic optician. However, a number of antibiotics are formulated in preparations for the eye and are frequently prescribed by medical practitioners. They include the following.

CHLORAMPHENICOL

This has a broad spectrum of activity and is often the drug of choice until the specific cause of the ocular infection is known. It is available as 0.5 per cent drops (including single dose) and 1 per cent ointment.

TETRACYCLINES

These are a group of antibiotics having bacteriostatic activity against a wide range of bacteria. Available preparations include tetracycline 1 per cent and chlortetracycline 1 per cent eye ointments and oxytetracycline 0.5 per cent with polymyxin B eye ointment.

NEOMYCIN

This has a broad spectrum of activity. The sensitivity of *Pseudomonas aeruginosa* to this antibiotic varies but is never high. Neomycin is available in eye drops and ointment, 0.5 per cent and in single-dose units containing 0.5 per cent. It is also available in combination with other antibiotics, for example, polymyxin B.

POLYMYXIN B

The activity of this antibiotic is restricted to Gram-negative bacteria, including *Pseudomonas aeruginosa.* Preparations available for topical use normally contain polymyxin and other antibiotics, for example, neomycin or oxytetracycline.

The antibiotics listed above are commonly used in the local treatment of ocular infections. However, if the infection is severe or deep-seated systemic as well as topical treatment may be used.

The penicillins are of limited use in the treatment of ocular infections. In general their effectiveness is restricted to Gram-positive bacteria and there is a high incidence of hypersensitivity reactions. Low stability in aqueous solutions and poor absorption give low concentrations which are dangerous in terms of resistance development. The exceptions which find use in the treatment of ocular infections are benzylpenicillin in gonococcal infections in the newborn and carbenicillin (systemically) in the treatment of Pseudomonas infections.

9

Solutions used in Contact Lens Work

Some of the solutions discussed will be used only by the contact lens practitioner during fitting; others will also be used by the patient in routine handling and care of the lens. The latter group will be considered first.

When inserted the lens should be free from contamination of any sort and it should be wettable.

Cleanliness

A contact lens may be contaminated with soaps, nicotine, fats, oils, cosmetics, dead skin and microorganisms which may be transferred to the lens during handling. Other contamination may arise from the mineral salts of tap water or protein, or oily and sebaceous secretions from previous wearings.

Wetting

Hard contact lens are made from polymethylmethacrylate and other ester polymers of methacrylic acid (*Figure 9.1a*). These have near ideal optical properties but they are hydrophobic and not easily wettable

(*a*)

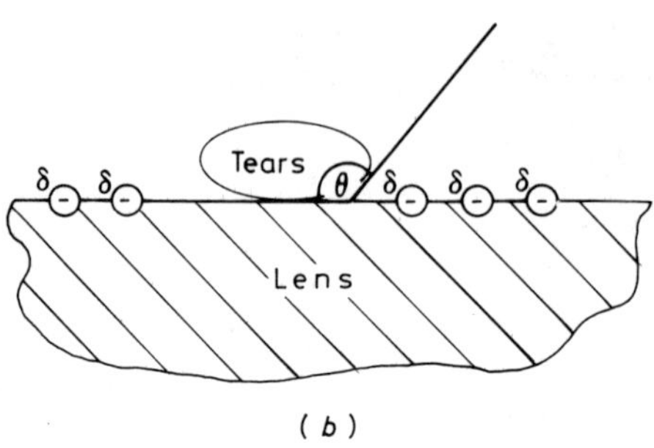

Figure 9.1 – Structure and wetting properties of polymethylmethacrylate: (a) subunit of the polymer polymethylmethacrylate; (b) angle θ for tears at the surface of a polymethylmethacrylate lens. (The high value of angle θ indicates that tears will not spread across the surface of the lens.)

(*Figure 9.1b*). If the lens cannot be wetted then it will be uncomfortable to wear. It is possible with the use of certain solutions to convert the outer layer of the lens to a hydrophilic one.

As the soft acrylic lenses are themselves hydrophilic there is no necessity for a wetting solution.

Hard contact lenses

The above factors suggest that one or two solutions are required for the use and care of hard contact lenses: (1) a wetting solution to be used immediately prior to inserting the lens; (2) a soaking/cleansing solution in which the lens is stored to remove and prevent contamination and maintain the hydrated state.

WETTING SOLUTIONS

Many patients use saliva as a wetting agent, and although it is effective its use should be discouraged. It contains mineral salts and protein material and increases the risk of bacterial contamination. A wetting solution should have the following qualities.

(1) Sterile and able to prevent contamination (the contact lens wearer is probably more prone to corneal epithelial damage making bacterial and fungal invasion easier).

(2) Suitable for direct undiluted application.

(3) Harmless to the eye after long-term use.

(4) Harmless to the lens after long-term use.

(5) Compatible with any other solutions used.

(6) Preferably isotonic to avoid movement of fluid in or out of the cornea with the associated discomfort.

(7) The pH of the solution should be in the range 5 to 9 if the solution is not buffered, and close to 7.4 if the solution is well buffered.

Mechanism of action

The mechanism by which wetting agents achieve their effect is shown in *Figure 9.2.* At the surface of the lens solute molecules orientate so

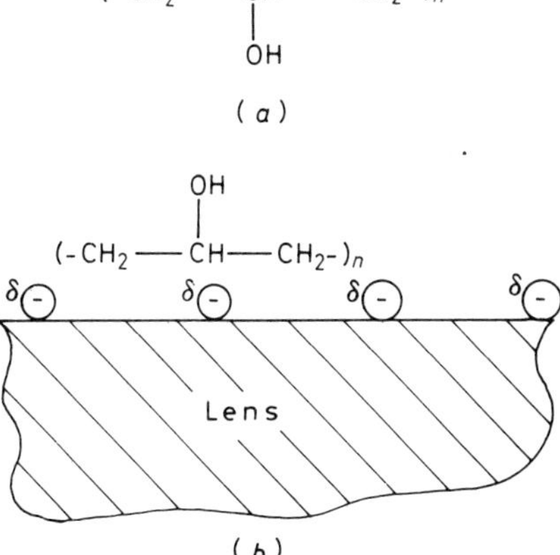

Figure 9.2 – Structure of polyvinyl alcohol and its orientation at a lens surface: (a) subunit of polyvinyl alcohol; (b) orientation of polyvinyl alcohol at the surface of the lens

that the hydrophilic end of the solute molecule is presented to the aqueous phase and the hydrophobic portion is presented to the hydrophobic plastic, this gives a hydrophilic interface and allows wetting of the plastic by the tears.

Advantages of wetting solutions

(1) They give the hydrophobic lens hydrophilic properties.
(2) The viscous solutions form a protective coating over the lens surface so that it does not come into direct contact with the finger during insertion. This will reduce the transfer of contaminants.
(3) They help stabilize the lens on the finger during insertion.
(4) They are an aid to cleansing after removal.
(5) They form a mechanical barrier between the lens and the corneal surface.

Composition of wetting solutions

Literature accompanying these proprietary preparations is usually incomplete and therefore precise details of the ingredients are uncertain. However, they are likely to contain polyvinyl alcohol and/or methyl cellulose. Polyvinyl alcohol is a wetting agent, it is non-toxic and non-irritant. Methyl cellulose is classed as a viscosity increasing compound, so it may not actually cause wetting. It has been reported to cause blurring of vision but it is non-irritant and does not cause tissue damage. There are also derivatives of methyl cellulose which may be used.

Wetting solutions also contain antibacterial compounds, for example, benzalkonium chloride, to reduce the risk of contamination during use.

Although benzalkonium chloride is a surface active agent it does not act as a wetting agent (*Figure 9.3*), it orientates with its hydrophilic portion towards the surface of the lens producing a new hydrophobic interface. Other antibacterial compounds may be used, including thiomersalate, chlorhexidine and phenyl mercuric nitrate.

SOAKING SOLUTIONS

Patients should be discouraged from using water, even if it has been distilled, because of the possible presence of chlorine, minerals and bacterial contamination. Water is hypotonic with respect to tear fluid and can lead to discomfort.

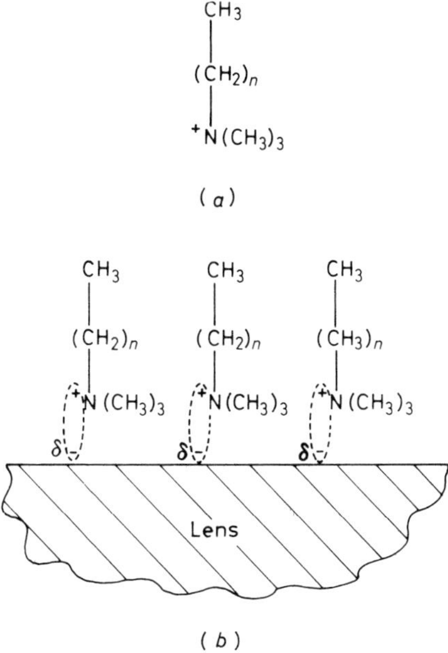

Figure 9.3 – Structure of benzalkonium chloride and its orientation at a lens surface: (a) subunit of benzalkonium chloride; (b) orientation of benzalkonium chloride at the surface of the lens

Soaking solutions should have the following qualities.

(1) Sterile and able to maintain the sterile state.

(2) Harmless to the eye.

(3) Harmless to the lens.

(4) Compatible with any other solutions used.

(5) Preferably isotonic.

(6) Of a reasonable pH in the range 5 to 9.

During wearing, protein, oily and sebaceous materials are deposited on the lens. If these are not removed they may collect in the micropores and reduce wettability and clarity. If these materials are allowed to dry on the lens a scum may be formed which is difficult to remove. During wear an equilibrium of hydration is reached which it is advantageous to maintain during storage.

Soaking solutions should therefore be capable of the following.

(1) Removing all secretions and deposits.

(2) Maintaining the state of hydration achieved during wear.

(3) Destroying any bacterial and fungal contamination, and preventing further contamination whilst the lenses are not being worn.

Composition

Most products contain one or more antibacterial agents, some may also have a chelating agent.

These are compounds which are able to complex with metal ions. After chelation the metal is no longer present as the metal ion and is unable to exert its normal actions. By this means it is possible to deprive bacteria of essential metal ions. The usual chelating agent is the disodium salt of ethylenediaminetetraacetic acid (disodium EDTA).

Soft contact lenses

An increasing number of people are wearing soft contact lenses. These soft acrylic lenses are hydrophilic and there is no need for a wetting solution. The material of the lens is more likely to concentrate any substance present in a soaking solution and this may then be released during subsequent wear. Therefore, the current practice generally is to avoid the use of conventional soaking solutions. It is recommended that the lenses be stored in isotonic saline solution. Manufacturers market a lens carrying/lens heating unit as a means of maintaining lens hygiene. The heating unit allows the lens to be heated to a temperature of 98–100°C over a standard period of time. It is claimed that this procedure eliminates most bacteria likely to contaminate the lens.

The remaining solutions are those used by the optician during fitting. They include local anaesthetics (Chapter 6), vasoconstrictors (Chapter 10), staining agents (Chapter 7) and antibacterial drugs (Chapter 8).

10

Decongestants, Antihistamines and Anti-Inflammatory Compounds

Decongestants

The drugs which are included in the sympathomimetic mydriatic group may also be used as decongestants. Peripheral blood vessels such as those present in the conjunctiva receive post-ganglionic sympathetic innervation. The activity of these nerves results in vasoconstriction due to the release of noradrenaline and its interaction with α receptors. Thus, adrenaline, phenylephrine and ephedrine will produce vasoconstriction when applied topically to the eye. The mechanisms by which they exert their effects have been discussed in the section on mydriatics. Compounds which are not used to produce mydriasis but which are used as ocular decongestants include naphazoline and xylometazoline hydrochloride. These are potent, directly acting, α receptor stimulants.

PREPARATIONS

Adrenaline solution

This may be prepared from either the tartrate or the hydrochloride salts giving a concentration of 0.1 per cent (1 in 1000) adrenaline. The solution may also contain chlorbutol and chlorocresol as preservatives, sodium metabisulphite as antoxidant and sodium chloride to produce an isotonic solution. The BP states that when adrenaline hydrochloride solution is prescribed adrenaline tartrate may be substituted. The solution should be stored in a cool place and protected from the light.

Phenylephrine and ephedrine

These substances may be used in solutions of the hydrochloride salt to produce vasoconstriction. A satisfactory decongestant action can usually be obtained with lower concentrations than those needed when a mydriatic effect is required. A concentration of phenylephrine, 0.25 per cent, has been recommended for use as a decongestant.

Naphazoline and xylometazoline

Naphazoline may be used as a decongestant in solutions containing 0.05 or 0.1 per cent. The solution should be adjusted to a suitable pH and tonicity. A preservative such as phenyl mercuric nitrate may be included and the solution should be stored protected from light. Xylometazoline is usually prepared as an 0.05 per cent solution in a formulation which also contains an antihistaminic drug.

USES OF DECONGESTANTS

These solutions may be used in contact lens work to prevent vasodilation which can occur during moulding and which would produce irregularities in the mould. The effects of adrenaline, 1 in 1000, usually last for less than one hour and may be followed by reactive hyperaemia. If vasoconstrictor solutions are used as decongestants to blanch reddened conjunctival vessels due to non-specific chronic irritation or allergy, the longer acting sympathomimetic drugs such as phenylephrine may be preferred. Prolonged use of vasoconstrictor agents is not to be recommended because of the danger of masking the symptoms of a more serious condition. With the longer acting drugs such as naphazoline the effect may last several hours, hence the rebound dilatation may be more marked.

Antihistamines

During an allergic reaction, for example, hay fever or hypersensitivity to atropine, it is thought that histamine and certain other substances present in tissues (5-hydroxytryptamine and various kinins) are released. Normally these substances are stored in a bound inert form but when released into the blood stream or extracellular fluid they affect tissues to produce itching, constriction of smooth muscle and vasodilatation. There is also an increased capillary permeability resulting in leakage of capillary contents and oedema. Thus, an allergic condition of the eye would present as a swollen, inflamed conjunctival area with severe itching and injection of the cornea. The ultimate remedy for this condition is the removal of the allergen. Temporary symptomatic relief of the condition may be achieved by the use of a vasoconstrictor (*see* above) and an antihistamine drug. The naturally occurring substance histamine will produce most of the signs of an allergic response when applied directly to the tissues. The antihistamine drugs compete with histamine for receptors in the tissue thereby antagonizing its actions. This antagonism is of the competitive type. The sympathomimetic drugs are not competitive antagonists but are described as 'physiological' antagonists. These drugs do not compete at the histamine receptor but produce vasoconstriction by a different mechanism, thereby reducing or abolishing the histamine vasodilation.

A preparation available to relieve the symptoms of an allergic condition of the eye contains antazoline sulphate (0.5 per cent) and xylometazoline hydrochloride (0.05 per cent). Benzalkonium chloride may be used as the preservative.

A large number of antihistamine drugs is available but are mostly formulated for oral administration used in the systemic relief of allergic conditions. Antazoline sulphate is chosen for use in the eye because it is less irritant to the eye than most other antihistamines applied topically.

Anti-inflammatory compounds

These drugs include the naturally occurring adrenocortical steroids and synthetic derivatives developed from the naturally occurring compounds. They are able to suppress and prevent all signs of inflammation, for example, redness and swelling, regardless of the initial cause. It is most important to note that steroids only prevent the signs of inflammation, they do not remove the underlying cause. Because of the danger of masking the development of serious systemic conditions the corticosteroids should only be used under medical supervision.

The systemic use of these compounds produces a number of undesirable effects including hypertension, oedema, electrolyte disturbance and hyperglycaemia. When used topically there is little danger of systemic effects.

The two most widely used preparations are hydrocortisone and prednisolone in the form of eye ointments or drops. They may be used by the medical profession for the symptomatic treatment of blepharitis, conjunctivitis and other local inflammatory reactions. The two main dangers associated with the topical use are a rise in intra-ocular pressure in some people predisposed to such an effect and cataract formation after long-term use. There is the danger that if the underlying cause of inflammation is bacterial, viral or fungal in origin then the infection may proceed even though the signs of its presence are suppressed.

11

Ocular Effects of Drugs Used Systemically

A high proportion of the people visiting the optician will be receiving systemic medication of some kind, with or without medical supervision. As some of the drugs may produce ocular effects it is necessary for the optician to be aware of these. Because the patients may not be able to name their drug treatment it is also necessary to know the conditions for which these drugs are routinely used. Thus, if the condition under treatment is known, the pharmacological group of drugs may possibly be deduced.

For some drugs an ocular effect can be predicted from their known pharmacological actions. For other drugs the ocular effect is not related to their major action but due to a minor aspect of their pharmacology. There is also a third group of drugs in which neither of the above situations apply, and the reasons for their ocular effects are obscure.

Drugs having possible ocular effects are shown in *Table 11.1*. The drug groups and their therapeutic applications are listed, together with the actions in the eye and an explanation of these actions, where known.

There are two important considerations in the use of the *Table*. First, not all the people receiving treatment with the drugs listed will show the ocular effects. Other considerations such as age and genetic factors may be important. Secondly, the list is not exhaustive, an abnormal drug response may be so rare as to have not received attention previously. Therefore, a practising optician may provide a service to the community at large if he is alert to the possibility that an ocular condition may be related to drug use (or abuse).

TABLE 11.1
Drugs capable of producing ocular effects after systemic administration

Condition treated	*Drug group and examples*	*Ocular effects*	*Explanation*
Cardiovascular			
(*a*) Hypertension	*Adrenergic neurone blocking agents*		
	Esbatal (Bethanidine)	Miosis	Removes sympathetic tone
	Declinax (Debrisoquine)	Ptosis	from iris and upper lid
	Ismelin (Guanethidine)		
	Noradrenaline depleters		
	Serpasil (Reserpine)	Miosis	Removes sympathetic tone
	Harmonyl (Deserpidine)	Ptosis	from iris and upper lid
	Rauwiloid (Rauwolfia)		
	False transmitters		
	Aldomet (Methyldopa)	Miosis	Removes sympathetic tone
	Hydromet (,, + Diuretic)	Ptosis	from iris and upper lid
	Ganglion blocking agents (rarely used)		
	Ansolysen (Pentolinium)	Cycloplegia	Removes dominant
	Inversine (Mecamylamine)	Mydriasis	parasympathetic tone from ciliary and sphincter muscles
Used also in other situations requiring diuretic action	*Thiazide diuretics*		
	Aprinox (Bendrofluazide)	Disturbed accommodation	Unknown
	Hydrosaluric (Hydrochlorthiazide)		
	Saluric (Chlorthiazide)		

TABLE 11.1 (cont.)

Condition treated	Drug group and examples	Ocular effects	Explanation
(*b*) Thrombosis	*Anticoagulants* Dindevan (Phenindione)	Disturbed accommodation	Unknown
(*c*) Heart failure Arrhythmias	Digoxin	Disturbed accommodation Disturbed colour vision Diplopia	May be central effect
	Quinidine (applies also to quinine used in other situations)	Disturbed accommodation Disturbed colour vision Photophobia Diplopia Constricted visual fields	Injury to retinal ganglion cells and nerve fibres? Retinal vascular changes?
Diabetes			
(*a*) Growth onset	Insulin	Corneal and lens oedema	Osmotic effect
(*b*) Maturity onset	*Oral hypoglycaemics* Rastinon (Tolbutamide) Diabinese (Chlorpropamide)	Disturbed accommodation	Unknown
Inflammatory conditions			
(*a*) May also be replacement therapy	*Corticosteroids* Hydrocortisone Prednisone Prednisolone Dexamethasone Betamethasone Triamcinolone	Cataract formation Rise in intra-ocular pressure	Unknown

TABLE 11.1 (cont.)

Condition treated	*Drug group and examples*	*Ocular effects*	*Explanation*
(*b*) May also be in malaria	Avlochlor (Chloroquine)	Disturbed accommodation Diplopia Retinopathy	Accumulates in the iris and choroid. Precise mechanism not known
Infections	*Sulphonamides*		
	Urolucosil (Sulphamethizole)	Disturbed accommodation	Unknown
	Septrin (Sulphamethoxazole + trimethoprim)		
	Batrim („ „ + „ „)		
	Others		
	Streptomycin	Optic neuritis	Unknown
	Streptotriad (Streptomycin + sulphonamides)		
	Isoniazid	Optic neuritis	Unknown
	Myambutol (Ethambutol)	Visual loss	Unknown
Epilepsy	Epanutin (Phenytoin)	Disturbed accommodation Diplopia Nystagmus	Central effect
	Tridione (Troxidone) Paradione (Paramethadione)	'Glare' phenomenon Disturbed colour vision	Retinal effect
Parkinson's disease	*Atropine-like drugs*		
	Artane (Benzhexol) Cogentin (Benztropine) Disipal (Orphenadrine)	Cycloplegia Mydriasis Photophobia	Removes parasympathetic tone from ciliary and iris sphincter muscles

TABLE 11.1 (cont.)

Condition treated	*Drug group and examples*	*Ocular effects*	*Explanation*
Ulcer	*Atropine-like drugs* Buscopan (Hyoscine) Merbentyl (Dicyclomine) Probanthine (Propantheline)	Cycloplegia Mydriasis Photophobia	Removes parasympathetic tone from ciliary and iris sphincter muscles
Allergy, Hay fever	*Antihistamines* Anthisan (Mepyramine) Fabahistin Histryl Piriton Tavegil and many more	Cycloplegia Mydriasis Photophobia	Possess some atropine-like activity May also be central effect
	Decongestants Triogesic Rinurel and many more	Mydriasis	Sympathomimetics stimulate iris dilator muscle
C.N.S. disturbances (*a*) Severe anxiety	*Phenothiazine tranquillizers* Largactil (Chlorpromazine) Moditen (Fluphenazine) Sparine (Promazine) Stemetil (Prochlorperazine) and many more	Acute: Cycloplegia Mydriasis Photophobia	Possess some atropine-like activity Also central?
		Chronic: Pigmentation of sclera and conjunctiva. Granular deposits in iris and cornea	Unknown
(*b*) Mild anxiety, nervous tension	*Anxiolytics* Librium (Chlordiazepoxide) Valium (Diazepam) Serenid-D (Oxazepam)	Disturbed accommodation	Possibly central effect

TABLE 11.1 (cont.)

Condition treated	*Drug group and examples*	*Ocular effects*	*Explanation*
(*c*) Depression, including mixed anxiety-depression	*Anti-depressants* Tryptizol (Amitryptyline) Tofranil (Imipramine) Surmontil (Trimipramine) and many more	Cycloplegia Mydriasis Photophobia	Possess definite atropine-like activity
	Limbitrol (Amitryptyline + Librium)	Cycloplegia Mydriasis Photophobia	Possess definite atropine-like activity
	Monoamine oxidase inhibitors Nardil	Disturbed accommodation	Unknown
(*d*) Motion sickness	*Atropine-like drugs* Kwells (Hyoscine)	Cycloplegia Mydriasis Photophobia	Remove parasympathetic tone from ciliary and iris sphincter muscles
	Phenothiazines Avomine (Promethazine)	Cycloplegia Mydriasis Photophobia	Possess atropine-like activity
	Antihistamines Dramamine Marzine	Cycloplegia Mydriasis Photophobia	Possess atropine-like activity

12

First Aid and Emergency Measures used by the Ophthalmic Optician

As opticians are not allowed to treat conditions of the eye first aid by the optician should be only what the words 'first aid' imply. That is, the measures taken should be sufficient to minimize any harmful processes and reduce the discomfort of the patient, then if necessary the patient should be referred to a doctor or the accident unit of a hospital.

The problems commonly met by the optician include the following.

Foreign bodies

If foreign bodies are easily removed it is permitted to do so using a cat gut loop or other suitable implement. A local anaesthetic instillation may make this task easier. A sterile fluorescein preparation to check for the presence of abrasions, and the prophylactic application of an antibacterial substance may be required. If the foreign body has penetrated the ocular tissues referral is essential. When a local anaesthetic is used care must be taken that the loss of the blink reflex does not expose the patient to the danger of further damage due to undetected foreign bodies. Therefore, the patient may be detained until the blink reflex has returned, or if this is not possible the eye could be covered with a pad. If both eyes have received local anaesthetic instillations some protection may be afforded by the instillation of some lubricant drops, for example, castor oil which is now available in sterile, single-dose, disposable containers, or liquid paraffin.

Other injuries

If the ocular tissues have received severe cuts, bruises or similar injuries it is necessary to refer the patient to a doctor.

Harmful chemical agents

LIME (QUICK LIME, CALCIUM OXIDE)

In the case of lime burns it is necessary to wash the eye as quickly as possible with water or sterile isotonic saline solution using a local anaesthetic to aid this if necessary. Some authorities recommend that washing should be continued for as long as thirty minutes. After this any adherent particles should be removed. If available a 10 per cent solution of ammonium tartrate may be used which will aid the removal of the particles. The chelating agent sodium edetate may be substituted for the ammonium tartrate.

SULPHURIC AND OTHER MINERAL ACIDS

In the case of acid burns to the eye immediate and prolonged washing with water or sterile isotonic saline solution is necessary. If available, sodium bicarbonate eye lotion may be applied but any advantage over water is minimal.

CAUSTIC SODA AND OTHER CAUSTIC SOLUTIONS

In the case of burns with alkaline solutions irrigation with a large volume of water or sterile isotonic saline solution is necessary. If available, citric acid eye lotion or a saturated boric acid solution may be necessary.

AMMONIA

Ammonia burns of the eye should be treated by washing with water or sterile isotonic saline solution. The washing may be followed by the instillation of liquid paraffin drops. In severe cases the anterior chamber may need draining because of the destructive effects of absorbed ammonia on the vitreous humour and retina. This procedure obviously is not first aid and referral is essential in such severe cases.

In most emergencies due to chemical injury the main safeguard is a mass irrigation of the eye which produces dilution of the offending agent, or physical removal in the case of non-water miscible liquids. In all cases where damage to the ocular tissues is suspected or where there is a risk of infection medical attention should be obtained immediately following the first aid measures.

13

Formulation of Eye Preparations

The preparations to be considered are eye drops, eye ointments and eye lotions.

Eye drops

When formulated and prepared, eye drops should contain the drug in such a form that it is well absorbed from the corneal surface and stable in the formulation. The solution should be sterile (and have some means of maintaining sterility). The ingredients of the eye drops should be compatible with each other and should not interact with the container or fastener. Attention may also be given during formulation to the tonicity of the solution. Isotonicity is preferable although not essential. The pH of the solution should be as near neutrality as possible.

ABSORPTION OF THE DRUG

This has been discussed at some length in Chapter 2 and the Appendix. Important factors for absorption are the pH of the solution and the pKa of the drug. If it is necessary to use a pH markedly different from neutral, then the drops may not be well tolerated by the patient. There may be stinging, irritation and probably loss of solution due to excessive tear production. Some authors suggest that most solutions between pH 3.5 and 10.5 can be tolerated. It is possible to aid the penetration of drugs by including in the formulation a wetting agent such as benzalkonium chloride. Wetting agents aid penetration by lowering surface tension and increasing the permeability of the membrane.

STABILITY

Since drops are not usually freshly prepared they must be formulated so that the active drug has a reasonable shelf life. Several factors may increase the rate of deterioration, for example, oxidation, pH, light, heat and hydrolysis.

Oxidation

A number of drops, for example, physostigmine are oxidized to yield products which may be less active and irritant. The oxidation process may be reduced by including in the formulation an antoxidant. Antioxidants are compounds which are preferentially oxidized. The antoxdant commonly used in eye preparations is sodium metabisulphite.

pH

The stability of drugs will vary depending on the pH of the drops. These may therefore be buffered to improve the stability. Care must be taken to ensure that the modifications to improve stability do not result in an irritant solution. An example of a buffered preparation is adrenaline eye drops; these contain a borate buffer to give a final pH of 7.4.

Light

Many drugs are adversely affected by light which may act as a catalyst to oxidative and hydrolytic processes. Drugs which are susceptible in this way should be stored in dark containers (amber glass) preferably in a light-proof cupboard. Phenylephrine and physostigmine are drugs which come into this category.

Heat

Some drugs are unstable to high temperatures. This will prevent the use of autoclaving and possibly heating with a bactericide as methods of sterilization. In this case filtration or aseptic techniques may be necessary to ensure sterility. Cyclopentolate is an example of a drug unstable to heat. Proxymetacaine is unstable at room temperature if oxygen and light are present; therefore it must be stored in a cool place.

Hydrolysis

As eye drops are usually formulated in an aqueous medium hydrolysis is a common problem. The only solution is to select constituents which are not susceptible to hydrolysis. This is not always possible, for example, with the local anaesthetic group of drugs. Hydrolysis of a drug may be reduced by storing the drops cool and in the dark.

STERILITY

Eye drops should be sterile, and when they are prepared in multidose containers the vehicle employed should be bactericidal and fungicidal to minimize the risk of contamination during use.

STERILIZATION

The *BPC (British Pharmaceutical Codex)* lays down three methods of sterilization together with regulations for the treatment of apparatus and containers. Apparatus and containers should be thoroughly cleansed before use. The teats of eye droppers are cleaned and impregnated with a solution containing the bactericide and other preservatives which are to be included in the final preparation. They should be stored seven days in this solution prior to use to allow equilibration to occur.

Autoclaving

The drug is dissolved in the vehicle containing the bactericide and any other ingredients. The solution is clarified by filtration and transferred to the final containers. These are sealed so as to exclude microorganisms and autoclaved at 115°C, 10 lb in^2 pressure for 30 minutes.

Filtration

The drug is dissolved as for autoclaving but the solution is then sterilized by passage through special bacterial filters. After filtration the solution is transferred to sterilized containers using aseptic techniques; and the containers are closed so as to exclude microorganisms.

Heating with a bactericide

The drug is dissolved in the vehicle containing the bactericide. The solution is clarified by filtration and transferred to the final containers. These are closed so as to exclude microorganisms and the drops sterilized by maintaining at 98–100°C for 30 minutes.

Drops may be sterilized by any other method providing that the final product is identical in appearance, quality and composition with one prepared by the above methods. For any method used the final product must comply with the sterility tests laid down in the *BPC.*

PREVENTION OF CONTAMINATION

Eye drops will be sterile until the time they are opened, after which there is the danger of bacterial and fungal contamination. The formulation must be able to maintain the sterile state. Any bactericidal or fungicidal substance included in the formulation must be: (1) effective at room temperature or below; (2) non-irritant and non-toxic; (3) compatible with the drug, other substances and containers; and (4) stable.

The *BPC* recommends three substances for use as preservative agents. They are: phenylmercuric nitrate or acetate, 0.002 per cent; benzalkonium chloride, 0.01 or 0.02 per cent; and chlorhexidine acetate, 0.01 per cent.

These three substances are chosen because they are effective (within limits), non-irritant, non-toxic and stable. The final choice of preservative is governed by its compatability with the active drug in the formulation and the purpose for which the drops are to be used.

PHENYLMERCURIC NITRATE, ACETATE

This possesses both antibacterial and antifungal activity. Although its activity against *Pseudomonas aeruginosa* is not very marked it is the best of the three recommended preservatives and the agent of choice for fluorescein drops. The antibacterial activity is unaffected by changing pH but it may be reduced by the presence of anionic agents. The solution should be protected from light. There is the possibility that metallic mercury may deposit on standing. It should not be used in drops such as pilocarpine which are intended for long-term use as there is the danger of mercurialentis. Sensitization may occur to phenyl mercuric nitrate. As a preservative in eye drops a concentration up to 0.002 per cent is used.

BENZALKONIUM CHLORIDE

This is a cationic surface-active agent. It is an effective bacteriostat and bactericide which is active against a wide range of Gram-negative and Gram-positive bacteria although the action against *Ps. aeruginosa* is rather slow.

By virtue of its surface-active properties benzalkonium reduces surface tension and causes changes in membrane permeability. These changes allow vital enzymes and other cell constituents to leak out of the cell. At the concentration used it is well tolerated by the eye, causing no irritation. Benzalkonium is incompatible with some anions including nitrate, salicylate, fluorescein and sulphonamides. The solution should be protected from light. As a preservative for eye drops it is usually used in the concentration 0.02 per cent. Benzalkonium will also aid penetration of the cornea by drugs, this may be useful in the case of carbachol, or undesirable for local anaesthetics.

CHLORHEXIDINE ACETATE

This is active against Gram-negative and Gram-positive bacteria with some activity against *Ps. aeruginosa*. It is unaffected by cationic compounds but is incompatible with anionic substances, for example, fluorescein. It should be protected from light and not allowed to come into contact with cork as this causes inactivation. Chlorhexidine acetate is usually used as a preservative in eye drops at a concentration of 0.005 to 0.01 per cent.

CETRIMIDE

This is a cationic quaternary ammonium compound with an activity similar to benzalkonium chloride. It may be used for preserving eye drops at a concentration 0.005 per cent. It may also be used for cleansing skin and in contact lens work.

THIOMERSAL

This has a similar action to phenylmercuric nitrate. It is bacteriostatic and fungistatic and is active against *Ps. aeruginosa*. For preserving eye drops it may be used at 0.01 to 0.02 per cent. The precautions and incompatibilities are the same as for phenylmercuric nitrate.

CHLORBUTOL

This is usually bacteriostatic and active against Gram-negative and Gram-positive organisms. It will inhibit the growth of *Ps. aeruginosa* at 0.5 per cent and is also active against fungi. It is stable to autoclaving at pH 6 or less but above this pH hydrolysis is increased by heat. It should be protected from light. A 0.5 per cent solution is close to saturation point and crystals may deposit at low temperature.

CHLOROCRESOL

This is a potent bactericide. It is used at 0.03 to 0.05 per cent when it is predominantly bacteriostatic. Some people may find this concentration painful on instillation. The solution should be protected from light.

TONICITY

At one time isotonicity was considered desirable even if not of prime importance. Many eye drops are hypertonic and this may cause stinging on instillation. Hypertonicity can only be corrected by dilution which would result in dilution of the active drug, usually below its effective concentration. Hypotonic solutions may be adjusted to isotonicity by the addition of sodium chloride.

CONTAINERS

The *BPC* lays down specifications for eye drop containers. Glass bottles should be amber, vertically ribbed (easily distinguished by touch from bottles with preparations for internal use), and made of neutral or soda glass provided that it has been treated to reduce the amount of alkali leached out by aqueous solutions (suitable plastic applicators may be used if they are capable of closure to exclude microorganisms). These containers should be fitted with a phenolic plastic screw cap. The cap incorporates a dropper of neutral glass and a teat of natural or synthetic rubber. Teats should be able to withstand autoclaving, and should not release alkali or other harmful substances. Silicone rubber is preferred if benzalkonium chloride is used as this reacts with the fillers used in the preparation of rubber. Alternatively, a complete dropper closure may be sterilized and supplied separately in a sealed package. In this case the bottle is closed with a plain phenolic plastic screw cap fitted with a suitable liner. The closure on bottles should be covered by a readily breakable seal.

Factors to be considered in the use of multidose containers

Whilst eye drops in multidose containers are prepared with a preservative there is always the danger of contamination with resistant organisms or the accumulation of dead bacterial cells and their contents. Therefore, in an attempt to minimize this the *BPC* has made recommendations as to how long a multidose container should remain in use after opening. For home use a period of not longer than four weeks is recommended and eye drops supplied for home use should carry a label to this effect, unless there are other special storage recommendations. For hospital wards a separate container should be provided for each patient, and for each eye if both eyes are being treated. They should be discarded not later than one week after first opening. In outpatient clinics and casualty departments opened containers should be discarded at the end of the day. Any patient who has undergone outpatient surgery should be treated with a separate supply of drops.

In operating theatres single-dose containers should preferably be used. If only multidose containers are available a previously unopened container should be used for each patient.

Eye drops of the *BPC* are not intended for introduction into the anterior chamber during surgery. Drops for this purpose should be sterile but contain no preservatives.

An obvious way to avoid contamination is the use of sterile single-dose disposable containers. These contain a small quantity (0.3 ml) of sterile fluid (sterilized by autoclaving at 115°C for 30 minutes) in a sterile plastic container. Not only are they sterile and disposable, thereby avoiding contamination, but they contain no preservatives. This lessens the likelihood of irritation and there is not the complication of incompatibilities in formulation. They may be preferable also for wearers of soft, acrylic contact lenses as these lenses are known to concentrate some preservatives, possibly leading to ocular irritation. Although these may be more expensive than traditional forms of presentation they offer the advantages of sterility, stability and an increased shelf life. The range available includes: atropine (1 and 2 per cent), homatropine (1 and 2 per cent), cyclopentolate (0.1, 0.5 and 1 per cent), hyoscine (0.2 per cent), ephedrine (5 per cent), phenylephrine (10 per cent), pilocarpine (1, 2, 3 and 4 per cent), amethocaine (0.5 and 1 per cent), oxybuprocaine (0.4 per cent), fluorescein (2 per cent), rose bengal (1 per cent), sulphacetamide (10 and 30 per cent) and neomycin (0.5 per cent).

Eye ointments

These contain the drug in a greasy base and are intended for application to the conjunctival sac or lid margin. The ointment is prepared from sterile ingredients using aseptic techniques. All apparatus to be used must be thoroughly cleansed and sterilized. In all cases the drug is incorporated in the following eye ointment basis: yellow soft paraffin, 80 per cent; liquid paraffin, 10 per cent; and wool fat, 10 per cent.

All the above ingredients are heated together and the molten base passed through a coarse filter paper into a clean container, the whole is then maintained at 160°C for one hour to ensure sterility. There are two methods of drug incorporation.

(1) As the base contains wool fat it absorbs water (up to 10 per cent). Thus, if the drug is water-soluble the sterile drug is dissolved in the minimum quantity of water and the solution sterilized by autoclaving or filtration and incorporated gradually in the melted sterile basis by aseptic technique. The finished ointment is transferred to the final sterile container which is closed so as to exclude microorganisms.

(2) If the drug is not water-soluble but soluble in the ointment basis the sterile medicament is finely powdered and thoroughly mixed with a small portion of the sterile melted basis. This mixture is incorporated with the rest of the sterile melted basis and transferred to the final container which is closed so as to exclude microorganisms. If the drug is not soluble in water or the basis, then it must be extremely finely powdered before incorporation to avoid irritation to the eye. After preparation the ointment must comply with the sterility tests of the *BPC*. Eye ointments contain no preservatives (bacterial or otherwise);

however, it is difficult for bacteria to survive in non-aqueous conditions, therefore contamination is unlikely. There is little possibility of oxidation or hydrolysis. When the ointment is supplied for home use the patient should be told to avoid contamination. The ointment should be applied direct from the container.

In hospitals and clinics separate containers should be used for each patient.

CONTAINERS

These are small collapsible tubes of suitable metal or plastic or suitable single-dose containers. Containers should be as free as possible (consistent with good manufacturing practice) from dirt and particles of the materials used in their manufacture. Tubes, caps and wads should be sterilized before use, cork wads are undesirable as they may harbour fungal spores. The container should be closed with a screw cap covered with a readily breakable seal or the whole tube enclosed in a sealed plastic envelope.

Eye lotions

These are sterile aqueous solutions to be used undiluted in first aid. These are of two types, as follows.

(1) Sterile aqueous solutions containing no bactericide for first aid or other purposes over a maximum period of 24 hours.

(2) Aqueous solutions containing a bactericide used for intermittent domiciliary use for up to 7 days.

The information on preparation and the standard for sterility applies to (1).

The *BPC* recommends that the apparatus used in their preparation and final containers should be thoroughly cleansed before use. The medicament is dissolved in water, clarified by filtration and transferred to the container. This is closed to exclude microorganisms and sterilized by autoclaving. Alternatively, the solution may be sterilized by filtration, transferred to the final sterile containers and then closed to exclude microorganisms. Not more than 200 ml should be supplied in a container. Lotions should comply with the sterility tests of the *BPC*. No preservatives are added, lotions are intended for short-term use only.

Lotions are also used for self-medication and are available in many proprietary forms. Some of these contain preservatives and may be used over a more prolonged period. Indiscriminate use at home should be discouraged as the use of a lotion may give temporary relief of ocular symptoms which require medical attention.

CONTAINERS

These should be coloured, fluted glass bottles. There should be an impermeable closure which must not contain cork, and be covered by a readily breakable seal. The use of non-fluted or colourless bottles is permitted if the fluted bottles are unavailable.

A number of eye lotions were included in the *BPC, 1963* but were subsequently deleted. The only one remaining in *BPC, 1973* is sodium chloride.

SODIUM CHLORIDE

The eye lotion contains 0.9 per cent sodium chloride in water and is isotonic with plasma. This lotion may be used in any situation where irrigation of the eye is required.

The large scale deletion of eye lotions from official publications is probably a reflection of the low esteem in which they are held.

14

Legal Aspects of Sale and Supply of Drugs

A number of the preparations used by the ophthalmic optician contain substances which are potentially dangerous. It is not desirable that these substances should be freely available; their supply, therefore, is restricted to people who have a legitimate requirement for such substances. The requirement may be one of use in a trade or profession, for example, that of optician, or it may be to treat an illness when the supply is made to a member of the public on a prescription of a registered doctor, dentist or veterinary surgeon.

At the time of going to press various provisions of The Medicines Act, 1968 are being brought into force to repeal the Pharmacy and Poisons Act, 1933. When the 1968 Act is fully effected all those parts of the Pharmacy and Poisons Act, 1933 remaining unrepealed will be repealed and replaced by the Poisons Act 1972. It is not expected that these changes will significantly modify the legal requirements and restrictions which currently apply to the ophthalmic optician. Therefore, the procedures involved in the sale and supply of drugs are likely to remain the same.

There are various acts of parliament which provide such a limited access to drugs, and they include the following.

The Pharmacy and Poisons Act, 1933 (soon to be repealed).

Misuse of Drugs Act, 1971.

The Therapeutic Substances Act, 1956 (on dates to be declared by orders under The Medicines Act, 1968 this act will be repealed and replaced by provisions in and under the 1968 Act).

The Medicines Act, 1968.

The Poisons Act, 1972.

Pharmacy and Poisons Act, 1933

This Act, together with the Poisons Rules and Poisons List made under it, lays down the regulations for the sale and supply of poisons. 'A poison' for the purposes of the Act is anything included in the Poisons List. Substances excluded are not subjected to the restrictions of the Act regardless of how toxic they may be. Also included in the Poisons List are substances which are not necessarily toxic but which it is considered inadvisable to be freely available for use without medical supervision.

The determination of what should and should not be included in the Poisons List is aided by a statutory advisory committee known as the Poisons Board. The composition of the Board is at present laid down in the Second Schedule to the Pharmacy and Poisons Act, 1933, and includes five members appointed by the Pharmaceutical Society and representatives from other professions concerned with the use and handling of drugs.

The Home Secretary, on the recommendation of or after consultation with the Poisons Board, decides whether or not a new compound should be included in the Poisons List. If the drug is related to a group which is already controlled then it may automatically come under control, for example, a new barbiturate or derivative will be controlled because the List contains the entry: 'barbituric acid; its salts, derivatives of barbituric acid, their salts; compounds of barbituric acids, its salts, its derivatives, their salts with any other substance.' Or the new drug may belong to a pharmacological group which is controlled, for example, central nervous system depressants and stimulants. If the drug does not fit either of these cases it may not be included initially. However, the Home Secretary has the power after consultation with, or on the recommendation of, the Poisons Board to amend or vary the Poisons List by a Statutory Instrument. This happens regularly. For example, quinine has enjoyed a popular reputation as an abortifacient. It has recently been transferred to control such that it is supplied only on prescription. Previously the only requirement was that quinine should be sold by an Authorised Seller of Poisons (ASP), that is, a registered pharmacist carrying on a business which comprises the retail sale of drugs.

The Poisons List[1]

This sets out those chemicals which are poisons in the terms of the Pharmacy and Poisons Act, 1933. It is divided into Part 1 and Part 2.

PART 1

Poisons in Part 1 may be sold only by an Authorised Seller of Poisons from registered premises when the sale is effected by, or under the supervision of, a registered pharmacist (Pharmacy and Poisons Act, 1933). The poisons included in Part 1 are mainly medicinal.

PART 2

These poisons may be sold as above (that is, by an Authorised Seller) and also by Listed Sellers of Poisons, being unqualified persons registered with a local authority to sell such poisons from specified premises (s. 18, Pharmacy and Poisons Act, 1933). The poisons in Part 2 are mainly used not for the treatment of human ailments but for household, agricultural, horticultural and industrial purposes. For the poisons sold by a Listed Seller there may be further restrictions on the particular form in which a poison may be sold. These restrictions are set out in Schedule 5 of the Poisons Rules.

The Pharmacy and Poisons Act, 1933, and the Poisons Rules also prescribe to whom these poisons may be sold and that records of sales must be kept by the sellers.

Poisons Rules[2]

The poisons controlled by the Act are classified into Schedules (independent of the Parts 1 and 2 classification in the Poisons List). The schedules lay down details regarding the transport, supply, records, labelling, etc., appertaining to poisons. The main schedules of importance to the optician are Schedule 1 (SI) and Schedule 4 (S4). The inter-relationships of the Poisons List and the Poisons Rules Schedules are shown in *Figure 14.1*.

[1] The current Poisons List in the Poisons List Order 1972 as amended (SI. 1972 No. 1938, as amended by SI. 1974 No. 80, SI. 1974 No. 1556, SI. 1975 No. 1072 and SI. 1976 No. 979).

[2] The current Poisons Rules are in the Poisons Rules, 1972 (SI. 1972 No. 1939, as amended by SI. 1974, No. 81, SI. 1974 No. 595, SI. 1975 No. 1073 and SI. 1976, No. 979).

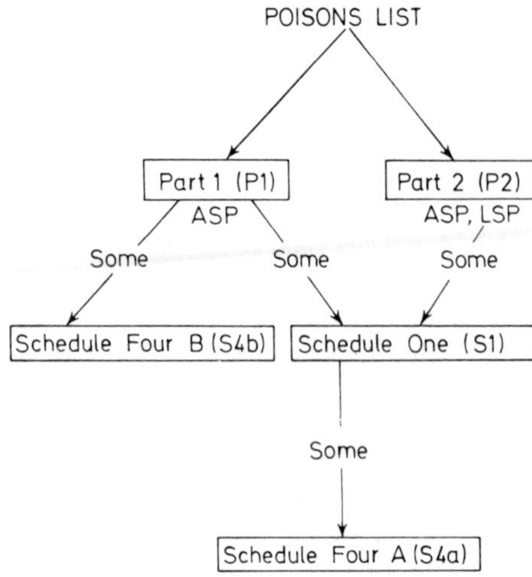

Figure 14.1 – Summary of Poisons List and Schedules

Availability of poisons to the optician

The availability and requirements to be met will depend on where in the List and Schedules the poison is included. If a drug is not included in the List it can theoretically be bought and sold by anyone, anywhere. However, in practice, it will be sold only by pharmacists and wholesale chemists. Eucatropine, cyclopentolate, lachesine and phenylephrine are drugs not included in the Poisons List and therefore fall into this category.

Poisons in Part 1 only

Ophthalmic preparations included in Part 1 only are: ephedrine eye drops and adrenaline eye drops.

One important point to note is that a poison may be included in Part 1 of the List only in one form, but in other forms or concentrations it may be included in the Schedules to the Rules.

For example,

ephedrine is:	Part 1 only	if in external preparations in which it forms less than 10 per cent of the

	solid preparation, or liquid preparations which are not aerosols.
Schedule 4	if in aerosol dispensers.
Schedule 1	in other cases.

Poisons in the First Schedule to the Rules (SI)

These are controlled as are poisons in Part 1 of the List but supply by retail is further controlled in that it can normally only be made according to one of the following ways.

(1) On the prescription of a duly qualified medical practitioner, registered dentist, registered veterinary surgeon or registered veterinary practitioner.

(2) In accordance with a signed order:

(*a*) if the person giving the order would normally use that poison in his trade or profession,

(*b*) if the person giving the order is engaged in that trade or profession at that time, and

(*c*) if the signature is believed to be that of the person giving the order.

(3) To a person known to the pharmacist and having a justifiable reason for requiring the poison.

(4) To a person unknown to the pharmacist but presenting a certificate signed by a householder known to the pharmacist guaranteeing that the intended purchaser is a person to whom the poison may be properly supplied.

(5) To a person unknown to the pharmacist presenting a certificate as in (4) signed by a householder unknown to the pharmacist and signed by a police officer in charge of a police station. Here the officer vouches for the reliability of the householder. The police officer gives no guarantee regarding the reliability of the intending purchaser.

The form of certificate required for (4) and (5) is set out in Schedule 11 of the Poisons Rules.

If the poison is supplied in accordance with (2), (3), (4) or (5) above the pharmacist must keep a record of the sale in his poisons book as set out in Schedule 12. The record must include the date of the sale, the name and quantity of the poison, the address and occupation of the purchaser, the purpose for which the poison is stated to be required, the date of any certificate, the name and address of any person giving a certificate and the purchaser's signature. In the case of a signed order the signature is not required for the poisons book entry.

An ophthalmic optician requiring a Schedule 1 poison for use in his practice, for example, physostigmine eye drops, could obtain a supply in one of two ways: (1) the poison could be purchased by the optician and the poison book signed as above; or (2) by the use of a signed order. A signed order should contain the following details:

(*a*) Name and address of purchaser.

(*b*) Profession.

(*c*) Name and quantity of poison or preparation required.

(*d*) Purpose for which required.

(*e*) Signature of the purchaser; this must be written and may not be printed or a rubber stamp used.

(*f*) Date.

A sample signed order is as follows.

Name ....

Address ....

....

Date ....

Please supply

1 × 10 ml Physostigmine Eye Drops BPC 1% for use in my profession.

Signature ....

Optician. FBOA

The pharmacist retains this order for a suggested period of two years and makes an entry in the poisons book as outlined above.

Poisons in the Fourth Schedule (S4)

The retail supply of Schedule 4 poisons is restricted to pharmacists, who may supply them only on prescription of a registered doctor, registered dentist, registered veterinary surgeon or registered veterinary practitioner. Any alternative supply can only be made to persons who by virtue of their trade or profession are specifically named in the

Poisons Rules as being exceptions to the primary restrictions. These special conditions for Fourth Schedule poisons apply to the optical profession. Thus, until recently, opticians could purchase Fourth Schedule poisons such as sulphacetamide eye drops for use in their profession. They could instil or administer such poisons but they were not authorised to supply these to their patients. Sulphonamides have recently been transferred from the Fourth Schedule of the Poisons Rules to control by the Therapeutic Substances Act (*see* later). Furthermore, orders for Fourth Schedule poisons given to patients by opticians are not valid unless they have been endorsed by a duly qualified medical practitioner. This restriction implies that the optician should only procure poisons of use in an optical practice. The Fourth Schedule is divided into parts A and B. Poisons in S4A, for example, demecarium bromide, are also in S1 and full records of the sale must be kept. Poisons in S4B are not included in S1 and therefore no records of the transactions need be kept. However, it is good practice for an optician to write a standard signed order for poisons in S4B, if he does not intend to present himself to the pharmacist.

There is generally no problem for the optician in obtaining the poisons he requires for his practice. The poisons required may be:

(1) Excluded from the Poisons List (cyclopentolate) and no restrictions apply.

(2) Included in Part 1 only, for example, amethocaine, and readily purchased from an Authorised Seller of Poisons.

(3) Included in the First Schedule, for example, atropine. Such poisons may be purchased from an Authorised Seller and the poisons book signed, or they may be obtained on a signed order.

(4) Included in both the First Schedule and Part A of the Fourth Schedule, for example, demecarium. Opticians are specifically allowed to obtain such poisons with a signed order.

(5) Included in Part B of the Fourth Schedule (until recently, sulphacetamide eye drops). Opticians are specifically allowed to obtain such poisons from an Authorised Seller.

One case which falls outside these situations may be met with. In order to obtain full cycloplegia in a young child an optician may decide that treatment with atropine eye ointment is required for several days. It is unnecessary for the child to return daily simply for application of the ointment. The optician cannot supply the ointment for home use (he is not an Authorised Seller of Poisons) and therefore must arrange for a supply for the child from a pharmacist. The recommended procedure is to give the child's parent a note to be taken to a pharmacist stating the name and address of the optician and containing a request that the pharmacist supply atropine eye ointment for application to the child's eye prior to refraction. The note should be signed and dated. A specimen note is given below.

Please supply to (name and address of patient)

1 × 3 G Atropine Eye Ointment BPC 1% for application to (child's name) eye prior to refraction.

Label: To be applied as directed.

Signed .... FBOA Optician.

The pharmacist may treat this situation in two ways:

(1) He may regard the optician's note as indicative that the poison is legitimately required. The supply may then be treated as a First Schedule sale. An entry is made in the poisons book with all the details and signed by the child's parent.

(2) Using the optician's note as evidence that the poison is legitimately required the pharmacist takes the responsibility and counter prescribes the atropine, making an entry in his prescription book.

If a supply is arranged and the preparation labelled without full directions (this is difficult on a 3 g ointment tube) then the optician must take care to give detailed instructions to the person who will be applying the ointment and be satisfied that the person understands and is capable of carrying out these instructions. As atropine is a toxic compound and produces effects in low concentrations a warning to this effect should be given. The following list includes some suggested advice and necessary precautions.

(1) An appropriate length (4–5 mm) of the tube's contents should be extruded into the lower fornix. This should be done twice daily for 3 days, but not on the day of refraction.

(2) Any excess ointment should be removed from the lids and lashes with cotton wool or paper towel, which should be burnt.

(3) The tube should be closed and stored in a safe place away from children.

(4) The hands of the person instilling the ointment should be washed.

(5) Precautions should be taken against transferral of the ointment from the recipient to other members of the family, for example, use of separate towel, etc.

(6) It should be stressed that the ointment is to be used only on the person for whom the supply was made. Any ointment remaining should be returned to the optician for disposal.

In the event of any untoward response (atropine irritation, or ingestion of the tube's content) the optician should be capable of recognizing the symptoms which would ensue (*see* pages 26–27) and taking appropriate action on referral.

Misuse of Drugs Act, 1971

This Act, and the Misuse of Drugs Regulations, came into force in July, 1973, and replaced the Dangerous Drugs Acts 1965 and 1967 and the Drugs (Prevention of Misuse) Act 1964. As the name implies, the Act deals with those drugs which are liable to misuse and, with some exceptions, capable of producing dependence. The drugs covered by the Act are the opiates (morphine, methadone, heroin, etc); the major central nervous system stimulants (cocaine, amphetamine); some minor stimulant drugs (for example, benzphetamine); the hallucinogenic drugs (for example, LSD – lysergic acid diethylmide); and cannabis. All these drugs are now known as Controlled Drugs. The Act makes the import, export, production, supply and *possession* of these drugs unlawful unless complying with the regulations of the Act. Thus, there are in the regulations specific classes of people who may lawfully possess Controlled Drugs. Ophthalmic Opticians are not specified; therefore they may not possess amphetamine, hydroxy-amphetamine or cocaine for use as either mydriatics, vasoconstrictors or local anaesthetics (in the case of cocaine).

Therapeutic Substances Act (TSA), 1956

This Act is divided into two parts as follows.

Part 1 controls the manufacture, labelling, packaging and importation of substances for medical use the purity or potency of which cannot adequately be controlled by chemical means.

Part 2 controls the sale, supply, dispensing and administration of penicillin and other antibiotics and certain hormones, for example, corticosteroids and their derivatives, and other substances capable of causing danger to the health of the community if used without proper safeguards. The sale or supply of Part 2 substances is restricted to a duly qualified medical practitioner, a registered dental practitioner or a registered veterinary surgeon or registered veterinary practitioner for the purposes of treatment by or in accordance with the directions of the practitioner or surgeon; *or* cases where the seller or supplier is a registered pharmaceutical chemist or an authorized seller of poisons (*see* above) and the substance or preparation is sold or supplied under the authority of a prescription signed and dated by such a practitioner or surgeon. The optician is not authorized to obtain a supply of these substances. Therefore the optician may not use steroids or antibiotic preparations. The propamidine derivatives and the compounds used as preservatives in eye drop solutions are not antibiotics and the Therapeutic Substances Act does not apply. Many of the antibiotics have a low toxicity and the Therapeutic Substances Act does not restrict the supply of antibiotics on this count. The main danger in improper use of antibiotics is the production of strains of bacteria which are resistant to the action of the antibiotic. Once resistance has developed there is the problem of finding a suitable alternative treatment, and in extreme cases no satisfactory alternative may be found.

The sulphonamides are not products of living organisms and therefore by definition (Chapter 8) are not antibiotics. However, because of their antimicrobial activity an amendment to the Therapeutic Substances Act transferred the sulphonamides from Schedule S4 of the Poisons Rules to Part 2 of the Therapeutic Substances Act. This made them unavailable to opticians for use in their profession. However, the Act has been further amended (October, 1972) allowing opticians specifically to obtain sulphacetamide and sulphafurazole eye drops or ointment for use in their profession.

Appendix

Passage of drugs across the cornea

The majority of drugs used by the optician are weak bases employed as their water-soluble acid salts. *Figure 2.1* shows ephedrine hydrochloride as a specific example. The general equation for the equilibrium between ionized and unionized forms of a weak base may be written as shown in *Figure A.1*.

$$\underset{\text{Ionized}}{RNH_3^+} + Cl^- \rightleftharpoons \underset{\text{Unionized}}{RNH_2} + H^+ + Cl^-$$

Figure A.1 – Dissociation of a weak base in solution

The ratio of ionized and unionized forms present in solution depends on two factors: the pKa of the drug, and the pH of the solution in which it exists. This ratio may be determined from the Henderson–Hasselbalch equation (*Figure A.2*). The pKa is an unchanging property

$$pH = pKa + \log_{10}\frac{[base]}{[acid]}$$

in this instance

$$pH = pKa + \log_{10}\frac{[RNH_2]}{[RNH_3^+]}$$

Figure A.2 – The Henderson–Hasselbalch equation

of the drug and is the pH at which it is 50 per cent ionized (that is, the concentrations of the ionized and unionized forms are equal).

Considering the example of a weak base pKa 9.4 (approximately that of atropine) prepared in a formulation of pH 6.4 as its acid salt. Then from the equation (*Figure A.3*) the ratio of the unionized to

$$6.4 = 9.4 + \log_{10} \frac{[RNH_2]}{[RNH_3^+]}$$

$$\log_{10} \frac{[RNH_2]}{[RNH_3^+]} = \bar{3}$$

$$\frac{[RNH_2]}{[RNH_3^+]} = \frac{1}{1000}$$

Figure A.3 – Calculation of degree of ionization of a weak base (pKa 9.4) in a solution at pH 6.4

$$7.4 = 9.4 + \log_{10} \frac{[RNH_2]}{[RNH_3^+]}$$

$$\log_{10} \frac{[RNH_2]}{[RNH_3^+]} = \bar{2}$$

$$\frac{[RNH_2]}{[RNH_3^+]} = \frac{1}{100}$$

Figure A.4 – Calculation of degree of ionization of a weak base (pKa 9.4) in a solution at pH 7.4

ionized will be 1:1000. If the pH surrounding the drug is 7.4, as in tears, the ratio will be 1:100 (*Figure A.4*). At the surface of the cornea the pH will be somewhere between 7.4 and 6.4 depending on the buffering ability of the tears. The proportion of the unionized form in solution will thus be somewhere between 1:100 and 1:1000. It is this unionized lipid-soluble form which crosses the epithelium.

Consider the equation (*Figure A.4*) where the base is one part in 100 parts unionized. When this one unionized part crosses the epithelium into the stroma, it will, itself, re-ionize according to the equation (*Figure A.5*). Assuming the pH in the stroma to be 7.4 the ratio of

$$RNH_3^+ \rightleftharpoons RNH_2 + H^+$$

$$\log_{10} \frac{[RNH_2]}{[RNH_3^+]} = \bar{2}$$

$$\frac{[RNH_2]}{[RNH_3^+]} = \frac{1}{100}$$

Figure A.5 – Calculation of degree of ionization of a weak base (pKa 9.4) in the stroma at pH 7.4

ionized to unionized will be 100:1. The ionized form, being water-soluble, will cross the stroma to the endothelium. Here a new equilibrium will be established between the two forms and the 1 part in 100 which is unionized will cross the endothelium into the aqueous.

The whole situation is a dynamic one and once any equilibrium is disturbed, as for example by the unionized form crossing the epithelium, the equilibrium will be re-established, in this case by dissociation of RNH_3^+. This will thus provide more unionized form to cross the epithelium, and again disturb the equilibrium. This re-establishment and disturbance of the equilibrium will take place at each of the three interfaces. In this way the drug will cross the cornea following a concentration gradient.

If a drug is completely ionized it will be unable to penetrate the epithelium. If the pKa of a weakly basic drug is low the ratio of unionized to ionized drug is high and there is therefore a higher proportion of this form available to cross the epithelium initially. A small change in pKa causes a large change in these ratios.

Figure A.6 shows the effect of changes in pKa in a series of local anaesthetic drugs. Thus, as the pKa rises from 7.9 for lignocaine through

	pKa	$\frac{[RNH_2]}{[RNH_3^+]}$ at pH 7.4
Lignocaine	7.9	1/3
Amethocaine	8.5	1/13
Procaine	8.9	1/32

Figure A.6 – The effect of changing pKa on the degree of ionization of a series of local anaesthetics at pH 7.4

8.5 for amethocaine, to 8.9 for procaine the ratio of unionized to ionized form in a solution at pH 7.4 changes from 1:3 to 1:13 to 1:32. Because of its higher pKa a larger proportion of the procaine molecule is ionized; conversely, because of its lower pKa a smaller proportion of the amethocaine molecule is ionized. This is one reason why procaine is less efficiently absorbed and therefore less effective as a corneal local anaesthetic.

The pKa of a drug cannot be changed but the pH of the eye drop formulation may be changed, within limits, to encourage a higher proportion of unionized drug at the cornea. Thus, as the pH of the formulation is raised the degree of ionization of a weak base will be reduced. The pH cannot be increased over the full range as too drastic a change from 7.4 (the usual pH of body fluids) will result in irritation of ocular tissues and possibly ocular damage. Changes in pH may also affect the solubility and stability of the drug. The pH must therefore strike a balance to give stability, reduced ionization and minimal irritation.

Index